Strength Training for Seniors

A Fitness Book for Seniors Offering Simple Exercises
to Boost Energy, Increase Muscle & Core Strength, Improve
Balance & Flexibility, and Build Confidence as You Age

Amy Neal

© Copyright 2023 - **All rights reserved.**

The content contained within this book may not be reproduced, duplicated or transmitted without direct written permission from the author or the publisher.

Under no circumstances will any blame or legal responsibility be held against the publisher, or author, for any damages, reparation, or monetary loss due to the information contained within this book, either directly or indirectly.

Legal Notice:

This book is copyright protected. It is only for personal use. You cannot amend, distribute, sell, use, quote or paraphrase any part, or the content within this book, without the consent of the author or publisher.

Disclaimer Notice:

Please note the information contained within this document is for educational and entertainment purposes only. All effort has been executed to present accurate, up to date, reliable, complete information. No warranties of any kind are declared or implied. Readers acknowledge that the author is not engaged in the rendering of legal, financial, medical or professional advice. The content within this book has been derived from various sources. Please consult a licensed professional before attempting any techniques outlined in this book.

By reading this document, the reader agrees that under no circumstances is the author responsible for any losses, direct or indirect, that are incurred as a result of the use of the information contained within this document, including, but not limited to, errors, omissions, or inaccuracies.

Thank you for buying my book! As a small token of my gratitude, here is a Quick Guide to Injury Prevention for Seniors. Just take a picture of the QR code with your phone, and you will receive the free PDF!

If you want to connect with me, find me at:

amynealcoaching.com

or on Facebook at:

Amy Neal Coaching

To my parents:

This book is dedicated to my mom and dad, my ultimate Senior Strength clients! I got into personal training when I was in my early 20's and my mom was one of my first trial clients! She was only in her 50's and was more than willing to let me try new workout ideas on her! She was always so supportive of me! My dad is who got me into fitness in the first place. He was my first bike riding buddy, kick ball buddy and when I got into softball, he was my throwing buddy! (Every single night!) My dad has always led by example in his health and fitness and always made being active, fun.

Training the two of them since 2017 has been one of the biggest joys of my life. To help keep them healthy, strong and active as they reach their mid 70's is such a good feeling. I smile when people say my parents are in such great shape, because with me being their daughter, they really didn't have a choice! I'm so thankful they made working out with me a priority.

Mom and Dad, thank you for your love and support my whole life! I love you both so much!

Table of Contents

Introduction 15

Chapter 1: The Importance of Muscle 17

    What Is Muscle? 17

    What Happens to Muscles During the Aging Process? 18

    Why Is Strength Training Important for the Elderly? 18

    The Physical Benefits of Strength Training for Seniors 18

    The Mental Benefits of Strength Training for Seniors 19

    The Social Benefits of Strength Training for Seniors 20

    Strength Training for Longevity 20

    How to Maintain Strength as You Age 21

    Myths and Misconceptions About Exercise and Aging 22

Chapter 2: Define Your Goals 23

    Why Fight Muscle Loss? 24

    Exercise Fights Brain Aging 25

    Healthy Antiaging Goals 25

    How to Set Health Goals and Stick to Them 26

    The Joy of Having Health Goals and Achieving Them 27

Chapter 3: Pick Your Program 29
    What Will the Exercise Program Entail?..29
        Resistance for Strength 29
        Stretching for Flexibility and More 30
    Which Muscle Groups Should I Train? 31
    I Don't Want to Be Sore After Exercising! 31
    I Have a Health Condition, Can I Still Exercise? 32
    Assessing Your Current Fitness Level 33
    Equipment for Your Home Exercise Program 34
    Timing...34
    When Should I Avoid Training? 35

Chapter 4: The Importance of a Good Warm-Up 37
    Why Should We Warm Up?...37
    Why Do We Stretch When Warming Up? 38
    Can I Finish With Stretching? 38
    Different Warm-Up Exercises 38
        Warming Up the Feet and Ankles 39
        Hip Flexor Stretching 39
        Leg Stretching 39
        Neck Stretching...39
        Sideways Back Stretching 40
        Glutes and Hip Stretching..40
        Quadriceps Stretching 40
        Hippie Stretch for Hamstrings and Lower Back 40
    Chair Warm-Ups...40
        Stretching the Achilles Tendon 40
        Shoulder Rolls 41
        Toe Taps..41
        Tummy Twist 41
        Seated Forward Bend 41
    Stretches for Warm-Ups and Daily Flexibility Routines..42

Simple Hamstring Stretch 42

Cat/Cow 42

Child's Pose 42

Overhead Side Stretch 43

V-Sit Stretch 43

Chapter 5: Functional Movements 45

What Are Functional Movements? 45

Squat 46

Variations for the Mobility-Impaired 47

Press Exercises 48

Shoulder Press 48

Bench Press 49

Seated Anchored Chest Press 49

Variations for the Mobility-Impaired 50

Push Exercises 50

Variations for the Mobility-Impaired 51

Pull Exercises 52

Variations for the Mobility-Impaired 53

General Functional Exercises for the Mobility-Impaired 54

Chapter 6: Accessory Movements 57

Single-Leg Deadlift 57

Variations for the Mobility-Impaired 58

Single-Arm Bent-Over Row 59

Variations for the Mobility-Impaired 60

Reverse Lunge 62

Variations for the Mobility-Impaired 63

Split Squat 64

Variations for the Mobility-Impaired 66

Thruster 66

Variations for the Mobility-Impaired 68

Chest Press on the Ground With Dumbbells 68
    Variations for the Mobility-Impaired 69

Bicep Curls 70
    Variations for the Mobility-Impaired 71

Box Dips 72
    Variations for the Mobility-Impaired 73

Lateral Raise 73
    Variations for the Mobility-Impaired 74

Hip Bridge 75
    Variations for the Mobility-Impaired 76

Kettlebell Swing 77
    Variations for the Mobility-Impaired 78

Plank 79
    Variations for the Mobility-Impaired 80

Side Plank 81
    Variations for the Mobility-Impaired 82

Leg Lifts 82
    Variations for the Mobility-Impaired 83

Chapter 7: At-Home Workouts 85

  Are Home Workouts Better Than a Gym? 86

  At Home Workouts: 86

  Lower Body Workout 1 87
    Warm-up: 87
    Strength: 87
    Finisher: 88

  Lower Body Workout 2 88
    Warm-Up: 88
    Strength: 88
    Finisher: 89

  Lower Body Workout 3 89
    Warm-Up: 89

 Strength: 89

 Finisher: 90

Lower Body Workout 4 90

 Strength: 90

 Core: 90

 Finisher: 91

Upper Body Workout 1 91

 Warm-Up: 91

 Strength: 91

 Finisher: 92

Upper Body Workout 2 92

 Warm-up: 92

 Strength: 92

 Finisher: 93

Upper Body Workout 3 93

 Warm-Up: 93

 Strength: 93

 Finisher: 94

Upper Body Workout 4 94

 Warm-Up: 94

 Strength: 94

 Finisher: 95

Full Body Workout 1 95

 Warm-Up: 95

 Strength: 95

 Finisher: 96

Full Body Workout 2 96

 Warm-Up: 96

 Strength: 96

 Finisher: 97

Full Body Workout 3 97

    Warm-Up: 97

    Strength: 98

    Finisher: 98

Full Body Workout 4 98

    Warm-Up: 98

    Strength: 99

    Finisher: 99

Using the Daily Workout and Healthy Habits Log 100

Chapter 8: Nutrition and Healthy Habits 103

Nutrition 103

    A Little More About Nutrients 104

Timing of Meals and Snacks for Optimal Performance 105

Hydration 106

Sleep 107

Amy's Advice 108

Chapter 9: Maintaining Strength and Avoiding Injury 109

The Importance of Consistency in Strength Training 109

The Importance of Consistency to Maintain Your Exercise Routine 110

Get the Most Out of Your Workout 110

Common Exercise Mistakes That Can Lead to Injury 111

Recovery and Rest 112

    Rest for Muscle Repair and Growth 112

    Rest for Reduced Risk of Injury 113

    Rest for Improved Performance 113

    Rest for Mental Health 114

    Rest for Hormonal Balance 115

Maintain Your Motivation 116

Overcoming Time and Energy Challenges 117

Social Support for Strength Training 118

Accountability 118

Chapter 10: Building Strength and Endurance............121

Progressive Overload and How to Increase Intensity Gradually 121
Importance of Proper Form 122
Incorporating Cardiovascular Exercise to Improve Endurance............122
Advanced Techniques for Strength Training 123
Plyometric Exercises............124
Plyometric Exercises for the Mobility-Impaired............124
Supersets............125
Supersets for the Mobility-Impaired............125
Isometric Exercises............126
Isometric Exercises for the Mobility-Impaired............127
Eccentric Training for Seniors............127
Eccentric Exercises for the Mobility-Impaired............128
Resistance Band Exercises 129
High-Intensity Interval Training............129
HIIT Exercises for Seniors............130
HIIT for the Mobility-Impaired............130
Overcoming Plateaus in Strength Training............131
Using Wii for Strength Training............132
Future Directions in Strength Training for Seniors 133
The Future of Strength Training for the Mobility-Impaired 134
Strength Training Games for Seniors............135
Strength Training Sports for Seniors............136
Aquatic Strength Training 136

Conclusion 139

References 143

Introduction

Aging is inevitable. As our bodies age, we get aches and pains, become weaker, struggle to walk upright, and have to guard against dreaded hip fractures. We have to stop doing what we love, be safe and sit still all day, and avoid physical activity to keep from getting hurt. Isn't this the sensible path to longevity? Amy Neal, speaking from years of experience as a certified personal trainer and nutrition coach, says no. There is a better way. She offers a path that leads to increased strength, increased confidence, and increased independence.

Amy isn't your typical trainer. She has been active in the fitness world since 2002 as a personal trainer and as a group trainer since 2013. Her clients, all with various abilities, range in age from 3–78. She specializes in strength training for women over 40 and has a particular passion for her Senior Class Strength Training. Seniors of every level of fitness have benefitted from her expertise and dedication. Teaching people about the benefits of strength training brings her joy that stems from the knowledge that she can genuinely help others to discover and maintain a healthier, more positive path in their golden years.

This book is a result of her personal experience of what works. She has participated in sports all her life, focusing on track and field. Her participation in sports while at school and college taught her the value of hard work and discipline, which fuels her dedication as a personal trainer. Her expertise and passion will help you achieve all the benefits of strength training in your senior years, resulting in a better quality of life, longevity, and the energy to enjoy every day to the fullest.

In this book, Amy will introduce you to the miracle of muscle. She explains why muscle is important and what role it plays in our bodies. She discusses what happens to muscles during the aging process and what benefits strength training can bring to seniors. Amy will inspire you and help you define your goals and decide on the where and when for your exercise program. Her knowledge will guide you through warm-ups, functional movements, and accessory movements. She includes 12 basic workouts that can be done in the comfort and privacy of your own home. Amy also lends her experience as a nutrition coach to explain key points about nutritional demands and healthy habits as we age.

This book provides guidance on how seniors can safely and effectively incorporate strength training into their exercise routines. Amy will lead you through detailed explanations and illustrations of various exercises that can be done with minimal equipment as well as provide information on proper form and technique.

The author addresses common concerns that seniors may have about strength training, such as the risk of injury and the need for modifications for those with medical conditions or physical limitations. Amy also included variations of exercises for people with limited mobility. Overall, this book presents strength training as a valuable tool for developing a healthy lifestyle that will help you live a long, active, independent life.

Chapter 1:
The Importance of Muscle

What Is Muscle?

Strength training is all about muscle. Before we start the exercises, let's take a look at what exactly we are exercising.

When muscle cells (myocytes) band together, they form muscle fibers. The three types of muscle cells in the human body are cardiac, skeletal, and smooth. The cardiac (heart) and smooth (lining the insides of our veins, arteries, stomach, and intestines) are involuntary muscles, which means they aren't consciously controlled and are regulated by the autonomic nervous system.

The skeletal muscles allow us to move. These are the muscles that we hear about in the gym or read about in fitness magazines, such as the biceps, hamstrings, calves, rectus abdominis (abs), and pectorals. They work in pairs; when one muscle contracts, the other elongates. Muscles are attached to bones by tendons. There are about 639 muscles in the human body. Some people have unique accessory muscles, which are natural variations in anatomy.

The largest muscle is called the gluteus maximus (the buttock muscle) and is responsible for hip extension. Hip extension is the movement that facilitates walking, standing, and running. The gluteus maximus is often shortened to "glutes." The smallest muscle, the stapedius, stabilizes the smallest bone (the stapes in the inner ear). Muscle is miraculous. From the largest to the smallest, from autonomic to consciously controlled, muscles enable us to explore, interact with, and enjoy the world.

What Happens to Muscles During the Aging Process?

The natural aging process causes muscle atrophy, which is the loss of muscle mass and strength, resulting in muscle weakness. This progressive atrophy is called sarcopenia. Sarcopenia can affect the musculoskeletal system by increasing frailty, which may lead to falls and fractures. We naturally start losing muscle in our 30s and 40s, and this loss rapidly increases around the age of 65, mainly due to hormonal changes, especially the lowering of testosterone and insulin-like growth factor (IGF-1) levels. It is estimated that you may lose as much as 8% of your muscle mass each decade (*Sarcopenia*, 2022). Sarcopenia is exacerbated by physical inactivity, obesity, chronic diseases (such as diabetes, chronic obstructive pulmonary disease, and cancer), malnutrition, arthritis, and inadequate protein intake. Sarcopenia symptoms include weakness, difficulty with balance, walking slowly, low stamina, and a decrease in muscle size.

Why Is Strength Training Important for the Elderly?

Resistance training geared toward developing strength is the best method to ward off muscle atrophy. Strength training contracts the skeletal muscle fibers to generate work against a given weight or external force. Muscles can be strengthened through the use of weight machines, free weights, resistance bands, and body weight. Strength training is easy and accessible, enabling the elderly to reap its benefits without having to travel to specialized clinics or buy expensive equipment.

Stronger muscles will help the older person remain independent for longer and be able to enjoy life. More strength and stamina will reduce the risk of falling, thereby also increasing confidence and the ability to take part in activities. Strength training may help ease symptoms of depression through the setting and achieving of goals. Exercise groups will curb the loneliness and feelings of isolation that the elderly often experience by providing social interaction and support.

The Physical Benefits of Strength Training for Seniors

Having a high quality of life and independence depends on how well we age. We have a greater measure of control over the aging process than many people know. With strength training, we can reverse and slow down the effects of time on our muscles.

- Strength training can rebuild up to four pounds of muscle after only four months of doing half-hour strength training sessions three days per week. This reverses the effects of sarcopenia.

- As we age, hormonal changes lead to more fat accumulation despite diet remaining the same. Since muscle is metabolically active and burns calories when in use, strength training will increase lean muscle and reduce fat. Strength training improves insulin sensitivity, which can drastically minimize the risk of developing type 2 diabetes when combined with healthy body weight and moderate fitness levels.

- Lower back pain is a common complaint as we get older, especially if we spend long hours sitting. Stronger muscles in the lower back can reduce this discomfort and ease the pain of arthritis and fibromyalgia.

- Strength training is heart-healthy! Nearly half of adult Americans have blood lipid levels that put them at risk of heart disease. A regular strength training regimen can reduce LDL (bad) cholesterol and triglycerides, and it can increase HDL (good) cholesterol by up to 23% (McKenna, n.d.). After only two months of strength training, resting blood pressure is lowered. Since hypertension (high blood pressure) is a risk factor for cardiovascular disease, the lowering of blood pressure reduces the chances of a heart attack.

- The musculoskeletal system includes muscle and bones, and thus strength exercises also benefit the bones. After several months of strength training, bone density increases and the risk of fractures decreases.

The Mental Benefits of Strength Training for Seniors

Strength training offers a wide range of mental benefits for seniors. Consistent resistance training is part of a good strategy for overall well-being.

- Strength training has been shown to boost the production of endorphins, which are natural "feel-good" chemicals in the brain. This can help relieve the symptoms of depression and anxiety and promote feelings of well-being and a positive outlook.

- Exercise, including resistance training, is a natural stress-buster. It helps reduce levels of the stress hormone cortisol in the body and can also increase the production and release of other neurotransmitters, such as serotonin and dopamine, which helps to promote a sense of calm and relaxation.

- Strength training can improve cognitive function and reduce the risk of progressive cognitive decline in older adults. It can help to improve memory, clarity, attention, and other cognitive abilities, which can have a positive impact on the overall quality of life.

- Strength training can help us feel stronger, more capable, and more confident in our abilities. This can translate into increased self-esteem and a greater sense of self-worth.

- Regular exercise, including strength training, can help induce deeper sleep and reduce the risk of insomnia. Better sleep can help improve mood, cognitive function, and overall quality of life.

The Social Benefits of Strength Training for Seniors

The social rewards of strength training will help you live a fuller, happier life. You'll have more fun and friends while experiencing less anxiety and loneliness. Increased strength and stamina will enable you to interact socially more, have more self-confidence, and be part of the fitness community.

- Participating in strength training classes or groups can provide you with opportunities for social interaction and engagement. You can meet like-minded people, make friends, and enjoy the camaraderie of working toward a common goal.

- As you improve your strength and physical abilities through strength training, you gain confidence in your abilities and feel more self-assured.

- Strength training has been shown to have positive effects on mental health, reducing symptoms of depression and anxiety.

As we age, we may become more isolated due to factors such as mobility issues or the loss of friends and loved ones. Participating in strength training can help us stay connected to others and maintain a sense of community.

Strength Training for Longevity

One study has found that independent of aerobic physical activity, adults over 65 who did strength training two to six times per week tended to outlive those who had less than two weekly training sessions, according to the author of the study, Dr. Bryant Webber of the US Centers for Disease Control and Prevention (LaMotte, 2022). Considering only statistical findings on strength training, the study found that adults who did four to six muscle-strengthening exercise sessions per week had a lower risk of death of any cause than adults who had less than two strength training sessions per week.

Here are some key ways strength training can impact longevity:

- As we age, our bones can become weaker and more prone to fractures. Strength training can help to maintain and even increase bone density, which will reduce the risk of fractures and osteoporosis. Fractures, especially of the hip and wrist bones, are common among the elderly and can take a very long time to heal.

- Muscle mass tends to decline with age, which can contribute to a range of health issues, including loss of mobility, insulin resistance, and metabolic disorders. Strength training can help preserve and even increase muscle mass, helping to maintain metabolic health and overall physical function.

- Falling is a major risk as we age and can lead to potentially serious injuries or even death. Strength training can help improve balance and mobility, reducing the risk of falls and promoting independent living.

- Strength training can help reduce the risk of a range of chronic diseases, including heart disease, diabetes, and certain types of cancer. By improving metabolic health and reducing inflammation, strength training can help promote a healthy immune system and reduce the risk of chronic disease.

How to Maintain Strength as You Age

Aging is inevitable, but the loss of muscle mass and strength is not. It is possible to maintain and even build muscle strength at any age. In a recent review of 14 studies of more than 500 healthy adults over the age of 65, resistance training was shown to be an effective method to improve muscle strength and performance in older adults suffering from sarcopenia (Hurst et al., 2022).

A healthy lifestyle helps us maintain strength as we age. Taking regular walks, doing cardiovascular exercises, and engaging in strength training help maintain healthy muscles (including the heart), boost energy, and improve balance and mood. A nutritious diet that limits alcohol and not smoking is part of a healthy way of life that contributes to well-being, longevity, and quality of life.

Myths and Misconceptions About Exercise and Aging

Myth: It's too late to start exercising as you get older.

Truth: It's never too late to start exercising. Even if you haven't exercised regularly in the past, you can still benefit from starting an exercise program. Exercise can help improve your overall health and reduce the risk of many chronic conditions. As long as you can move, you can exercise. If you have limited mobility, you may benefit from exercises that are adapted to your abilities.

Myth: As you get older, you should focus on low-intensity exercise.

Truth: While it's important to listen to your body and adjust the intensity of your exercise routine as you age, low-intensity exercise isn't the only option. High-intensity exercise can also be beneficial for older adults, as long as it's done safely and appropriately. Begin with low-intensity exercises and gradually build the intensity level.

Myth: Strength training is only for young people.

Truth: Strength training is important for people of all ages. Resistance training is particularly important for older adults as it can help maintain muscle mass, improve bone density, and reduce the risk of falls.

Myth: You can't build muscle or improve fitness as you get older.

Truth: While it's true that the aging process can make it more difficult to build muscle and improve fitness, it is still possible to make progress. Regular exercise can help maintain and improve strength, endurance, and overall fitness.

Myth: Older adults shouldn't do any high-impact exercise.

Truth: It is important to be mindful of the impact of exercise on your joints. Some keyed-down high-impact exercises can still be safe and beneficial for older adults. For example, low jumping and jogging can help improve bone density and overall fitness. Aquatic exercises are an effective alternative if you suffer from joint pain. Working out in water is easy on the joints while offering more resistance than air, which will improve muscle strength.

Chapter 2:
Define Your Goals

Starting anything new can be daunting, especially when we have reason to be afraid. If you have ever suffered from an injury due to a fall, the prospect of taking a walk or having an exercise routine may feel intimidating. If you recently had a health scare and know you must make a lifestyle change, you might feel overwhelmed and unsure of how to start or uncertain about what will benefit you. Perhaps you are starting to feel the aches and pains associated with getting older and want to strengthen your muscles to relieve discomfort but are afraid that exercise will cause even more pain. It is a big step, but the rewards are worth it.

I have seen the transformation that exercise can bring to the elderly. I am inspired by my friend Ivah who, at the age of 78, loves life, enjoys good food, and is active. Ivah wasn't actively participating in strength or fitness classes until her daughter threatened to make her come live with her on the other side of the country… unless she started weekly strength training. Ivah kept up her end of the deal and committed to a twice-weekly strength training program. I have trained her consistently twice a week for three years, only missing a session when she is traveling. She still lives a happy, independent life in her own home. It is exciting to see the gains in Ivah's strength and balance. Knowing that Ivah isn't at risk of falling or breaking a hip or wrist due to poor balance or posture, that her heart is strong, and that she is capable of living a full, independent life is comforting.

When Ivah started her strength training, she was aware that aging had slowed down her fitness level. She knew that she had to keep her goals realistic and easy to achieve. It is easier to progress with smaller goals that can be reached within weeks than to unrealistically think we can run a marathon with a month's training. Unrealistic goals can make us feel inadequate and cause us to abandon our training programs. Realistic goals reward us with pride in our achievements and encourage us to stick to our exercise routines. It's always amazing to see the progress Ivah makes!

Why Fight Muscle Loss?

One study has found that about 30% of adults over the age of 70 have trouble with ordinary tasks such as getting out of a car, walking, or climbing stairs (Freedman & Martin, 1998). Mobility limitations show a correlation to increased incidences of falls, admissions to nursing homes, chronic diseases, and mortality (*How Can Strength Training*, n.d.). Unfortunately, most people are unaware of the effects of age on our muscles, and they don't know that we can still have healthy muscles as seniors.

As we age, there are a number of changes that can occur in our muscles, collectively known as sarcopenia. Sarcopenia is the gradual and progressive loss of strength, muscle mass, and function that occurs with aging. Here are some of the ways that muscle changes as we age (*How Can Strength Training*, n.d.):

- Starting in our 30s, we begin to lose muscle mass at a rate of about 3–8% per decade. By age 75, we may have lost up to 30% of our muscle mass if we don't do resistance training.

- With age, the size of individual muscle fibers also decreases, which further contributes to the loss of muscle mass.

- As muscle mass and fiber size decrease, so does muscle strength. This can make it harder to perform everyday tasks like climbing stairs, getting into the bath, or carrying groceries.

- Our muscles and tendons become less flexible with age, which can increase the risk of injury and limit our range of motion. This is what causes us to feel stiff and achy.

- Aging muscles may tire more quickly, making it harder to sustain physical activity. We need more rest more frequently.

- Muscle recovery time increases with age, which can result in longer periods of soreness and fatigue following exercise or physical activity.

Age-related changes can have a significant impact on our overall health and quality of life; however, regular exercise, especially strength training, can help slow or even reverse some of these effects and promote healthy muscle aging.

Exercise Fights Brain Aging

Sticking to an exercise routine has several benefits for seniors, including improvements in cognitive health. Exercise can benefit cognitive health in older adults in the following ways:

- Exercise has been shown to improve memory and cognitive function in seniors. During exercise, blood flow increases, and more oxygen becomes available to the brain, which can enhance recall and other cognitive abilities.

- Regular exercise has been associated with an increase in brain volume in seniors, which helps to maintain cognitive function and prevent cognitive decline associated with aging.

- Exercise is a weapon against the risk of developing dementia in older adults. Research shows that regular exercise can reduce the risk of dementia by up to 50% (Alzheimer's Society, 2019).

- The brain also responds to exercise by improving executive function, which includes the ability to plan, organize, and prioritize tasks. This enables us to maintain our independence and perform activities of daily living more effectively.

- Anxiety lessens due to the relaxing effects of exercise. Exercise can also help reduce symptoms of depression in seniors. This can help improve overall mental health and cognitive function.

Overall, regular exercise can have a significant positive impact on cognitive health in seniors. You are never too old to start exercising, and even small amounts of physical activity can have benefits for cognitive function and overall health.

Healthy Antiaging Goals

Setting your sights on having a healthy lifestyle is the path to improved overall health, mobility, and more independence in your senior years. Building your goals around healthy habits will help you achieve and maintain healthy muscle aging. Here are some must-haves to include in your plans for a healthy lifestyle:

- Exercise is essential for building and maintaining muscle strength. Try to do at least 30 minutes of moderate exercises, such as walking or swimming, five days a week. Be consistent with your program.

- Include strength training exercises in your workout routine to build and maintain muscle mass. Using resistance bands or light weights will improve muscle strength and prevent muscle loss.

- Drinking enough water is essential for muscle health as it helps keep muscles hydrated and functioning properly. Avoid drinks that are high in sugar. Just because a liquid is called a sports drink doesn't necessarily mean that it is healthy.

- To maintain optimal health, we should consume a balanced diet that includes plenty of protein to support muscle growth and repair. High-protein foods include lean meats, fish, eggs, beans, and legumes.

- We need to get adequate sleep to help our bodies repair and regenerate muscle tissue. Your goal should be to get at least seven to eight hours of sleep each night.

- Stretching will improve flexibility and range of motion, which can help prevent falls and other injuries.

- Smoking and excessive alcohol consumption can harm muscle health and contribute to muscle loss. If you are a smoker, consider quitting. Talk to your doctor about methods you can use to help you kick the habit.

By using these tips for your daily routine, you can achieve healthy muscle aging and improve your overall quality of life.

How to Set Health Goals and Stick to Them

Setting health goals is an excellent way to improve your overall well-being, but sticking to them can be challenging. Here are some steps to help you set health goals and stick to them:

- Choose a health goal that is realistic and attainable. For example, if your goal is losing weight, start with a small goal of losing five pounds in a month. If you want to do 10 pushups, start by doing three. Once you achieve those goals, gradually move the goalpost further. If you set unrealistic goals, you will feel frustrated and be tempted to abandon your goals altogether.

- Keep a journal. Write down your goal and the steps you need to take to achieve it. Having a written plan can help keep you on track and accountable. This book contains a fitness log where you can write down the types of exercises you do as well as the number of repetitions and sets and your heart rate.

- Break your ideals down into bite-size pieces. Break your goal down into smaller, more manageable tasks. This makes the goal seem less overwhelming and more achievable.

- Decide on a timeline for each goal. Draw up a timeline with deadlines for each step. This helps you stay focused and motivated.

- Get support. Be sure to share your goals with people who will support and encourage you, such as family, friends, exercise groups, or even online support groups.

- Track your progress and celebrate when you reach a goal; doing so can help you stay motivated and on track. Reward yourself every time you reach a goal.

- Be prepared to adjust your goals as needed. Life happens, and it's essential to be flexible and make changes when necessary. It is better to change your goal than to resent the time spent exercising. You don't have to spend hours every day working out to experience the benefits.

- Staying positive and optimistic can help keep you motivated and focused on your goals. Be kind to yourself and celebrate your progress.

The Joy of Having Health Goals and Achieving Them

Having and achieving health goals can bring about many joys and benefits in one's life; here are some of them:

- Increased energy: When you eat healthier, exercise regularly, and take care of your body, you will naturally have more energy throughout the day. This can help you be more productive, feel less tired, and have more motivation to tackle your daily tasks.

- Improved mood: Performing regular exercise releases endorphins, which are naturally produced by the body to give it a feeling of well-being. Achieving your health goals can also bring about a sense of accomplishment and pride, which can improve your overall mood.

- Improved self-confidence: When you achieve your health goals, you may feel more confident in your body and your abilities. This can translate into other areas of your life, such as work, relationships, and social situations.

- Better sleep: Regular exercise and healthy eating habits can improve the quality and duration of your sleep, which allows you to feel more rested and alert during the day.

- Reduced stress: Exercise reduces stress levels by releasing tension in the body and calming the mind. Achieving your health goals can also reduce stress by giving you a sense of control and accomplishment in your life.

- Reduced risk of chronic diseases: By eating a nutritious diet, exercising regularly, and maintaining a healthy weight, you can reduce your risk of chronic diseases, such as heart disease, diabetes, and certain types of cancer.

Chapter 3:
Pick Your Program

Is it possible for a 75-year-old to build and maintain muscle, stay flexible, and enjoy bike riding? My own father is proof that it isn't just possible, it can be done at home without breaking the bank. My dad Mike decided about seven years ago that he would start strength training with me. He was an avid bike rider, and he realized that he needed to maintain and build muscle to keep enjoying his biking. As he's aged, he rides less, but he strength trains consistently twice per week. His balance, cardiovascular strength, and musculature are excellent. He works on his mobility daily at home and stays flexible. His commitment to showing up each week is very inspiring!

What Will the Exercise Program Entail?

Resistance for Strength

Resistance training is a type of exercise that involves using resistance, such as dumbbells, kettlebells, or resistance bands, to challenge and stress the muscles. This stress stimulates the muscles to adapt and become stronger over time. Resistance training can be an effective way for seniors to build strength, maintain muscle mass, and improve overall health. Here are some ways resistance training can build strength in seniors:

- The natural aging process can cause us to lose muscle mass and strength. Resistance training can help to counteract this by promoting muscle growth and increasing muscle size.

- Resistance training improves muscle function, such as the ability to produce force, contract quickly, and maintain force over time.

- Resistance training can increase bone density, which can help reduce the incidence of falls and fractures in seniors.

- Resistance training can increase the metabolic rate, which means the body burns more calories at rest. This can help seniors maintain a healthy weight and avoid the onset of chronic diseases such as diabetes.

- Resistance training can improve your balance and coordination, which can help to prevent falls and maintain independence in seniors.

Stretching for Flexibility and More

Including stretches in your exercise routine is a smart investment in your body. Here are the benefits of regular stretching:

- The aging process can cause our muscles and joints to become stiff and inflexible. Stretching can help maintain or improve flexibility, which can make it easier to perform daily activities, such as bending down to pick something up or reaching for an object on a high shelf.

- Stiff muscles and joints can increase the risk of falls and other types of injury. Stretching can help to improve the range of motion, reduce muscle tension, and increase blood flow to the muscles, all of which can reduce the risk of injury.

- Our balance and coordination can decline with age, which can increase the risk of falls. Stretching can help improve balance and coordination by reducing muscle imbalances and enhancing proprioception, which is the body's sense of where it is in space.

- Stretching can help alleviate pain and stiffness in the muscles and joints, which can be especially beneficial for seniors who suffer from arthritis or other chronic pain conditions.

- Regular stretching can also have mental health benefits as it can help reduce stress and anxiety, promote relaxation, and improve overall mood and well-being.

Which Muscle Groups Should I Train?

Strength training works by using resistance to challenge the muscle. There are several major muscle groups that are commonly targeted in strength training:

- The chest muscles, or pectorals, are responsible for movements such as pushing and pressing. Strengthening the chest muscles can improve upper body strength and posture. Good posture results in better balance and less pain in the back, shoulders, neck, hips, and knees.

- Back muscles, including the latissimus dorsi (at the side of your back) and trapezius, are responsible for pulling movements. Strengthening the back muscles can improve posture and reduce the risk of back pain.

- The shoulder muscles, including the deltoids and rotator cuff muscles, are responsible for movements such as lifting and rotating the arms. Strengthening the shoulder muscles can improve upper body strength and stability.

- Arm muscles, including the biceps and triceps, are responsible for bending and extending the elbows. Strengthening the arm muscles can improve grip strength and overall upper body strength.

- Abdominal muscles, including the rectus abdominis (the six-pack abs) and obliques, are responsible for stabilizing the core and supporting the spine. Strengthening the abdominal muscles can improve posture and reduce the risk of back pain.

- Leg muscles, including the quadriceps at the front of the thighs, hamstrings, and glutes, are responsible for movements such as squatting, jumping, and running. Strengthening the leg muscles can improve lower body strength, balance, and mobility.

I Don't Want to Be Sore After Exercising!

Soreness after exercise, also known as delayed onset muscle soreness (DOMS), is caused by microscopic damage to muscle fibers that occurs during exercise. This damage can lead to inflammation and the release of chemicals that stimulate nerve endings. This process may result in soreness, stiffness, and tenderness in the affected muscles. There are several strategies that can help reduce or avoid DOMS:

- Gradually increase the intensity of your workouts: Soreness is more likely to occur when you suddenly increase the intensity of your workouts. Instead, gradually increase the intensity over time to allow your muscles to adapt.

- Warming up and cooling down: Warming up before exercising and cooling down after can help prepare your muscles for exercise beforehand, help them recover afterward, and prevent injury.

- Stretching: Incorporating stretching exercises into your routine can help improve flexibility and reduce muscle soreness.

- Staying hydrated: Adequate hydration is important for proper muscle function and recovery.

- Getting enough rest: Getting enough sleep and allowing your muscles time to rest and recover is crucial for avoiding soreness and injury.

- Getting proper nutrition: Eating a well-balanced diet with sufficient protein and carbohydrates can help support muscle recovery and reduce soreness.

- Using recovery tools: Using tools like foam rollers, massage balls, and compression garments can help reduce muscle soreness and aid in recovery.

Remember that some degree of soreness after exercise is normal, especially when you're first starting a new fitness routine or changing up your routine. However, by gradually increasing the intensity of your workouts, taking steps to properly warm up and cool down, staying hydrated, and getting enough rest, you can help to minimize soreness and recover faster.

I Have a Health Condition, Can I Still Exercise?

Exercising with certain health conditions requires special considerations and modifications to ensure safety and effectiveness. Here are some tips for exercising with common health conditions:

- Arthritis: Low-impact exercises such as walking, swimming, and cycling are good options for those with arthritis. Resistance bands can be used to strengthen the muscles without putting stress on the joints. Avoid high-impact exercises that may exacerbate joint pain.

- Osteoporosis: Weight-bearing exercises, such as walking and weight lifting, can greatly restore bone density and reduce the risk of fractures. Exercises that involve bending or twisting the spine should be avoided.

- Heart conditions: Aerobic exercises, such as walking and cycling, can help improve cardiovascular health. It is important to start slowly and gradually increase the intensity and avoid high-impact exercises that may put too much stress on the heart.

- High blood pressure: Aerobic exercises, such as walking and swimming, can help reduce blood pressure. Resistance training can also be beneficial, but you should avoid holding your breath during exercises as this can cause blood pressure to rise.

- Parkinson's disease: Exercises that focus on balance and coordination, such as yoga and tai chi, can be beneficial for those with Parkinson's disease. Low-impact exercises, such as cycling and swimming, can also help improve mobility. When doing strength training, do the exercises seated and start with light weights.

- Diabetes: Aerobic exercises, such as walking and cycling, can increase insulin sensitivity and blood sugar control. Resistance training will also be beneficial. Seniors with diabetes should monitor their blood sugar levels and avoid exercises that cause pain or discomfort.

- COPD: Breathing exercises, such as pursed-lip breathing and diaphragmatic breathing, can improve lung function and reduce shortness of breath. Low-impact exercises, such as walking and cycling, can also be beneficial, but it is important to start by doing only a few light exercises and gradually increase intensity. Start your strength training by doing only as many repetitions as you find comfortable.

Assessing Your Current Fitness Level

Assessing your fitness level is an important step before starting a strength training program. It will give you a baseline idea of your current strength and balance levels and show you which areas you need to focus on. Here are some ways you can assess your fitness level for strength training:

- Visit your doctor: Before starting any exercise program, it is wise to consult your doctor, especially if you have heart conditions, osteoporosis, or conditions such as Parkinson's disease that affect your muscular control and balance. A doctor can evaluate any medical conditions or medications that may affect your ability to engage in strength training and recommend appropriate exercises.

- Perform a basic fitness test: You can perform a basic fitness test to evaluate your current fitness level. This can include tests such as a one-minute sit-to-stand test to evaluate leg strength, a 30-second arm curl test to evaluate upper body strength and a six-minute walk test to evaluate cardiovascular endurance.

- Consider balance and flexibility: In addition to strength, balance and flexibility are important components of fitness. You can assess your balance by performing a one-leg stand or walk test, and you can assess flexibility through tests such as the sit-and-reach or shoulder stretch.

- Start with light weights: If you are new to strength training, you should start with light weights and progressively increase the weight as you become stronger. Starting with light weights also reduces the risk of injury.

- Monitor progress: It is important to monitor progress over time to see improvements in strength, balance, and flexibility. Keeping a fitness journal or log, like the log provided in this book, can help you track your progress and adjust your workouts accordingly.

Equipment for Your Home Exercise Program

Dedicate a space in your home exclusively for your exercises. You don't need an entire room. A small space in your garage, a corner of a room, or a space on the back patio will do. It is important that the area where you are going to exercise doesn't have anything on the floor that you could trip over. You will also need a chair, a box or bench, small dumbbells, a set of light kettlebells, comfortable clothes, tennis shoes, and a mat or towel. As you get more comfortable with your home workouts, you can add equipment.

Timing

To reap the benefits of resistance training, two days per week is an adequate minimum. As you become stronger, you may need more training days to reach your desired outcomes. Here are three training options to help you achieve your goals:

- 2 days per week: 1 upper body day and 1 lower body day, or 2 full body days

- 3 days per week: 1 upper body day, 1 lower body day, 1 full body day
- 4 days per week: 2 upper body days and 2 lower body days, focusing on different body parts each day

When Should I Avoid Training?

It is ideal to exercise every day, but under certain conditions, it is sometimes wise to take a break. If you have to skip workouts, don't neglect your health goals. Stay on track by making sure you are hydrated, eating nutritious food, and getting enough sleep. Avoid training under the following conditions:

- If you recently had surgery or have surgery scheduled, consult with your doctor before you start or resume your exercise program.
- Don't exercise if you are in pain or have an injury. Wait until your injury has fully healed or your doctor advises you to exercise.
- Skip your workout if you have a fever, a contagious illness, or feel generally unwell. Get some rest and focus on recovery.
- Sometimes we have days where we feel more tired and exhausted than normal. If your body tells you to rest, skip your workout and take it easy.
- If you're experiencing sudden or severe pain during exercise, it's important to stop and seek medical attention. Continuing to exercise could make the pain worse and lead to further injury.
- Avoid exercising on very hot days to reduce the risk of dehydration and heatstroke. If you are exercising somewhere with air conditioning, you still have to make sure you're properly hydrated before, during, and after exercise.

Chapter 4:
The Importance of a Good Warm-Up

Meet my mom, Christine. She is 75 years old and has some health issues—a curved spine, nerve pain from the curved spine, arthritis, hip pain, and a meniscus tear—yet she consistently shows up for her workouts twice per week. She has been training with me for five years. Christine had to put her training schedule on hold when she had to have certain surgeries for her knee and foot, but she always returns to her training program as soon as possible. She knows she has to keep working her muscles, strengthen her core, and maintain good mobility. Her well-being and quality of life depend on it. She gets frustrated when she can't do what she thinks she should still be able to, but she still shows up. Whenever she goes to a doctor's appointment, they are impressed with how strong and flexible she is. Her doctors are always pleased with the results of her bloodwork. This is the result of consistency in strength training! She is amazing!

Why Should We Warm Up?

Warm-ups are essential to any workout, especially for seniors, to reduce the risk of injury. The warm-up prepares the body for the demands of the workout. Your body will warm up, your heart will beat faster, and your joints and muscles will become more elastic and less prone to tearing or spraining. The increased blood flow will make more oxygen available to the muscles during your workout. Your range of motion will be greater with warm muscles and tendons than without a warm-up.

Why Do We Stretch When Warming Up?

The warm-up stretch doesn't only prime our muscles for exercise—it also offers another benefit: It will help keep us flexible. Stretching exercises are crucial to maintaining and improving balance and core strength and preventing falls. Stretching and strength training go hand in hand. As we age, the connective tissue between our bones becomes less elastic, which reduces mobility, and our range of motion becomes smaller. Stretching reverses this process by elongating the muscles around the joints, keeping us mobile and reducing the risk of injury.

If you are planning to work out, incorporate some stretches into your warm-up routine. Stretch before and after your exercises to reap the full benefits. If it isn't a workout day, stretch in the morning and before bed.

Can I Finish With Stretching?

Stretching is an excellent cool-down exercise. Cool-down exercises are an integral part of any workout routine as they help your body transition from a state of intense activity to a state of rest. If you suddenly stop exercising, your blood pressure can fall too quickly, which can cause dizziness or fainting. Cool-downs will gently slow your heart rate and decrease your blood pressure. Incorporating cool-downs to round off your exercise routine will reduce the risk of injury, particularly to the muscles you worked during your session. Stretching during your cool-down session will help improve your flexibility and range of motion. To cool down properly, you can do stretches, walk, or jog gently.

Different Warm-Up Exercises

Many people neglect the warm-up part of the exercise routine. The warm-up is a crucial part of any exercise program, and it will get the body and mind ready for the workout that follows. These exercises are ideal warm-ups, suitable for the whole body. Remember to keep the spine straight during warm-ups, breathe deeply, and don't force yourself to stretch beyond your comfort zone. Keep your movements smooth and easy. If you find any movement painful, stop immediately. Choose the warm-up exercises that will target the same muscles that you plan to use in your workout.

Warming Up the Feet and Ankles

Loosen up your ankles and legs with the following warm-ups:

- Sit comfortably on a chair with your feet on the floor and hold your spine straight. Splay your toes outward 20 times. You don't have to hold the stretch. Don't rest in between the splays.

- Stand on one leg (hold on to something steady if you are a beginner or have balance issues). Rotate your foot 10 times clockwise and 10 times counterclockwise. Stand on the other leg and repeat the warm-up.

- Stand with your feet together. Keep your heels on the ground and lift the toes of one foot upwards in the direction of your knee. Hold the stretch for five seconds and repeat with your other foot.

Hip Flexor Stretching

The hip flexors are the muscles that allow us to lift our legs and bend at the waist. Warm them up with a stretching exercise that is done seated on a chair. Keep your back straight during this warm-up. Put the ankle of one foot on the opposite knee and bend forward from the hips. Hold this position for 20 seconds and repeat with the other foot.

Leg Stretching

Stand in front of a wall and hold your arms straight out to the front, a little lower than shoulder height. Put your hands on the wall and lean forward while keeping your feet flat on the ground. Stretch the calf muscle by standing on your heels for 20 seconds. Hold onto a steady object to avoid losing your balance when doing this exercise.

Neck Stretching

You can do this warm-up while seated in a chair or standing. Keep your shoulders held down and back while doing this exercise. Lower your chin to your chest to stretch your neck muscles. Hold your chin against your chest and move your left ear towards your left shoulder. When you have gone as far as you can comfortably go, hold the stretch for 20 seconds. Do the same with your right ear toward your right shoulder. Return your head to the middle and, with your chin still tucked, roll your shoulders backward 20 times.

Sideways Back Stretching

Stand upright with your feet hip-width apart and keep your arms at your sides. Bend your upper body to your left while keeping your lower body still. Hold the bottom of your bend for 20 seconds. Bend to the right for 20 seconds.

Glutes and Hip Stretching

Stand up straight with your feet shoulder-width apart; hold onto a stable object if you are a beginner or have balance problems. Keep your upper body as still as you can and swing each of your legs 20 times out to the sides.

Quadriceps Stretching

Stretch the muscles at the front of your thighs by standing up straight and holding onto something steady. Stand on one leg and bring the other leg's foot up behind you toward your glutes. Grab hold of that foot and hold the stretch for 20 seconds. Repeat this process with the other leg.

Hippie Stretch for Hamstrings and Lower Back

Stand with your feet together and flat on the ground. Slide your hands slowly down the front of your legs. Move your hands down only as far as is comfortable. If you push yourself further than a comfortable stretching sensation, you risk injury. When your hands are at the lowest part of the stretch, let your head hang loosely down. Hold this stretch for 30 seconds. If you feel dizzy, start by holding the stretch for only a few seconds and gradually add more time. An added bonus to the increase in flexibility is the feeling of releasing tension. You might feel more relaxed after doing this stretch.

Chair Warm-Ups

These warm-ups aren't just for people with limited mobility as they are suitable for everyone's exercise routine.

Stretching the Achilles Tendon

While sitting down, loop a towel, rope, or exercise band around the soles of your feet. Straighten your legs. You can stretch your ankles with your legs parallel to the ground, but you will also get results if you start with your heels on the floor and slowly straighten your knees. If you find ankle stretching challenging to do with your thighs parallel to the floor, keep your heels on the floor, slide your feet forward, and straighten your knees. Pull your rope toward your chest to stretch the Achilles tendon, which is behind the ankle above the heel. When your legs are straight, keep tension in the rope for 20 seconds. You can do both feet at once or each one separately.

Shoulder Rolls

Sit comfortably with your back and neck as straight as possible. Keep your feet on the floor and shrug your shoulders upward as if you want to touch your ears with your shoulders. Roll your shoulders 10 times in a clockwise direction and 10 times counterclockwise.

Toe Taps

To warm up, stretch, and strengthen the muscles of your lower legs, sit up straight with your feet flat on the floor. Keep your heels on the floor and lift your toes toward the ceiling as far as you can. Hold the stretch for five seconds and lower your toes back down. Repeat this exercise five times.

Tummy Twist

Sit comfortably upright and try to keep your back and neck as straight as possible. Tuck your elbows at your sides and hold your forearms straight out in front of you. Hold your lower body still and tighten your core muscles by pulling your belly button in toward your back. Turn your upper body as far as you can to the left and then to the right. Do 10 repetitions to each side. The tummy twist targets your obliques (the muscles in your abdomen that are used to rotate your upper body) and will improve your flexibility and posture.

Seated Forward Bend

To stretch your back, sit with your feet and knees a little wider than shoulder-width apart. Hold your feet flat on the floor during the entire exercise and lean slowly and smoothly forward. Your elbows will be on the inside of your lower legs and your hands will drop to the floor. Bend your upper body as far forward as you comfortably can and hold the stretch for 30 seconds.

Stretches for Warm-Ups and Daily Flexibility Routines

Simple Hamstring Stretch

The hamstrings are the muscles in the back of the thighs and can be stretched with a move we all know, the toe touch. Stand up straight and bend forward to touch your toes, or get as close as you comfortably can. Keep your legs straight during the stretch. When you have reached as close to your toes as possible, hold the stretch for 20 seconds. Not everyone can touch their toes when they start flexibility training. If you find it difficult, be patient and consistent, and you will find that you will eventually reach your goal.

As a variation, you can cross one foot in front of the other during this exercise. Bend at the hip, keep your legs straight, and let your head hang down to your knees. Stop immediately if you feel a straining sensation on your neck. Hold the stretch for 20 seconds. Repeat the hold with the other leg in front.

Cat/Cow

The cat/cow stretch is a floor exercise used by yoga practitioners as a stress reliever. Get on all fours with your knees under your hips and your arms straight out with your hands under your shoulders. Inhale slowly and deeply while you curve your lower back toward the floor and your belly drops. Tilt your pelvis up toward the ceiling and lift your head up. This is the cow part of the stretch. Follow the cow directly with the cat-like stretching motion. Exhale slowly and deeply while arching your back up toward the ceiling. Drop your head and pelvis towards the floor. Repeat the movements for one minute.

Child's Pose

Another stretch with relaxation and stress management as an added benefit is the child's pose. Kneel on the floor and sit on your heels with your knees held slightly apart. Keep your glutes on your heels during the entire stretch. Lean forward until your forehead touches the floor (you can put a pillow under your forehead for extra comfort). You can reach your arms out in front of you or have them stretched out behind you next to your legs, palms toward the ceiling. Hold this position for one minute while you inhale deeply and exhale as completely as you can.

Overhead Side Stretch

The overhead side stretch adds strength and flexibility to the muscles on your sides and the intercostal muscles, which are the muscles between your ribs. This stretching exercise can be done while standing or sitting. Keep your feet hip-width apart and your body facing forward during the entire stretch. Be aware of your posture to prevent your back and shoulders from hunching during the movements. With your right arm raised overhead, bend your upper body to the left. Hold the bend for 20 seconds and repeat with your left arm overhead bending to the right.

V-Sit Stretch

Sit on the ground with your legs held in a V shape (spread out). Reach in front of you between your legs as far as you can and hold the stretch for 30 seconds. Keep your spine neutral and reach toward your left foot, holding the stretch for 30 seconds. Repeat the reach toward your right foot and hold it for 30 seconds, and then return to the middle. If you are a beginner, start with only a few seconds and consistently add another second until you can hold the stretches for 30 seconds. If you are more advanced, you can add more time to your holds and gradually add more repetitions.

Don't swing your arms, because if you use momentum and not your muscles, you won't get the full benefits of this stretch. Your legs stay on the ground during the entire exercise.

Chapter 5:
Functional Movements

What Are Functional Movements?

Functional movements are the basic movements your body is capable of. Every exercise is a variation of these seven foundational movements. A functional movement uses large muscle groups that work together. When putting together an exercise routine, each functional movement has to be included at least once per week. Exercises based on functional movements resemble movements we would ordinarily make every day, such as picking up, carrying, or pushing an object. The purpose of functional movement exercises is to make it easier to do these regular movements we make during the day.

Squat

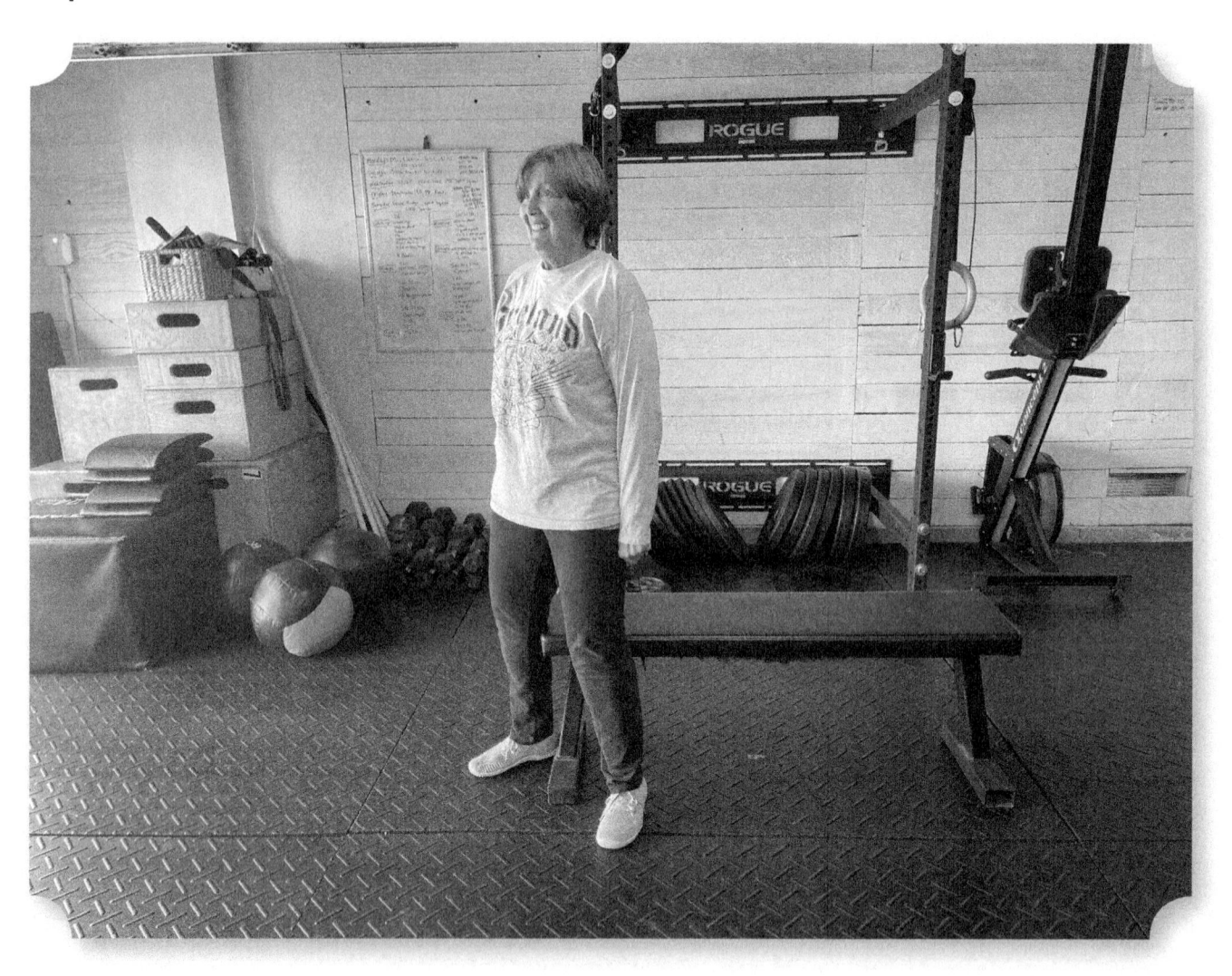

Functional squat exercises improve our balance and strength, making it easier to get up and down without falling. You become steadier and can get up out of a chair or sit down in the bath without losing your balance. Picking something up off the floor becomes painless and easy.

Stand with your feet about shoulder-width apart. Keep your head in a neutral position as tilting your head up might cause you to risk injury by arching your back. With both feet flat on the ground, push your glutes backward and lower them until your thighs are parallel to the ground. It is normal to lean slightly forward at the bottom of the movement but don't bend all the way over—try to keep your chest up. Lift yourself up by pushing up through your heels and straightening your knees and hips. You can extend your arms in front of your body to help keep your balance. If you are a beginner, start by doing three squats and add one more every week until you can do 10.

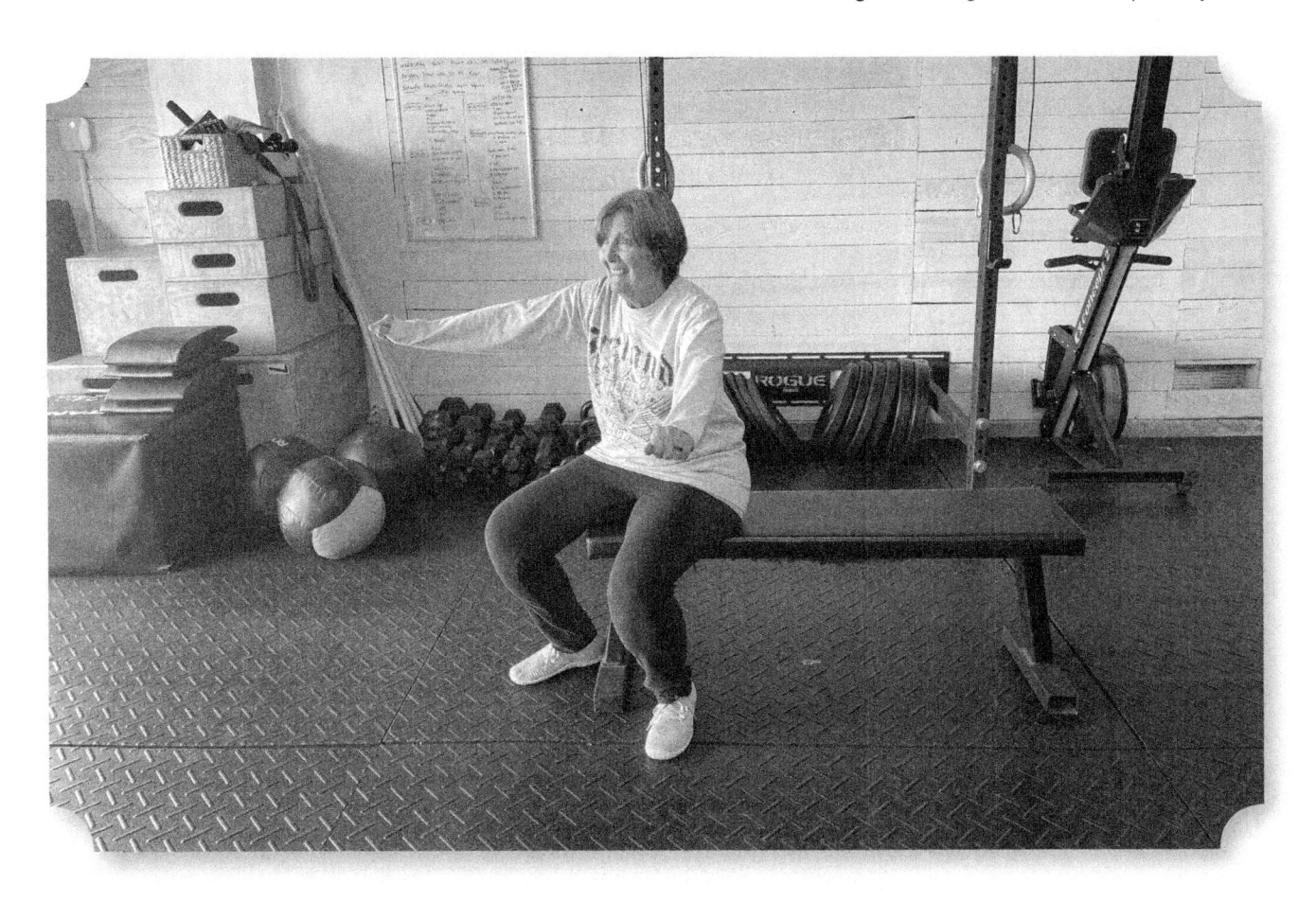

Variations for the Mobility-Impaired

When it comes to functional squat exercises for mobility-impaired seniors, it's important to choose exercises that are safe, effective, and easy to perform. Here are some exercises to consider:

- Sit-to-stand squats: This exercise involves sitting on a chair and standing up repeatedly. It helps strengthen the legs and improves mobility. Start with 1–2 sets of 10–12 repetitions and gradually increase the number of sets and repetitions as you get stronger.

- Wall squats: Start this exercise by standing with your back against a wall and then lowering yourself into a squatting position. This helps improve leg strength and balance. Start with 1–2 sets of 10–12 repetitions and gradually increase the number of sets and repetitions to keep challenging your muscles.

- Body weight squats: For this exercise, stand with your feet shoulder-width apart and lower your body into a squatting position. This exercise helps improve leg strength and balance. Start with 1–2 sets of 10–12 repetitions and gradually increase the number of sets and repetitions as your strength increases.

- Step-ups: To perform this exercise, step up onto a low platform or step, then step back down. This exercise helps improve leg strength and balance. Start with 1–2 sets of 10–12 repetitions on each leg and gradually increase the number of sets and repetitions as your strength improves.

Press Exercises

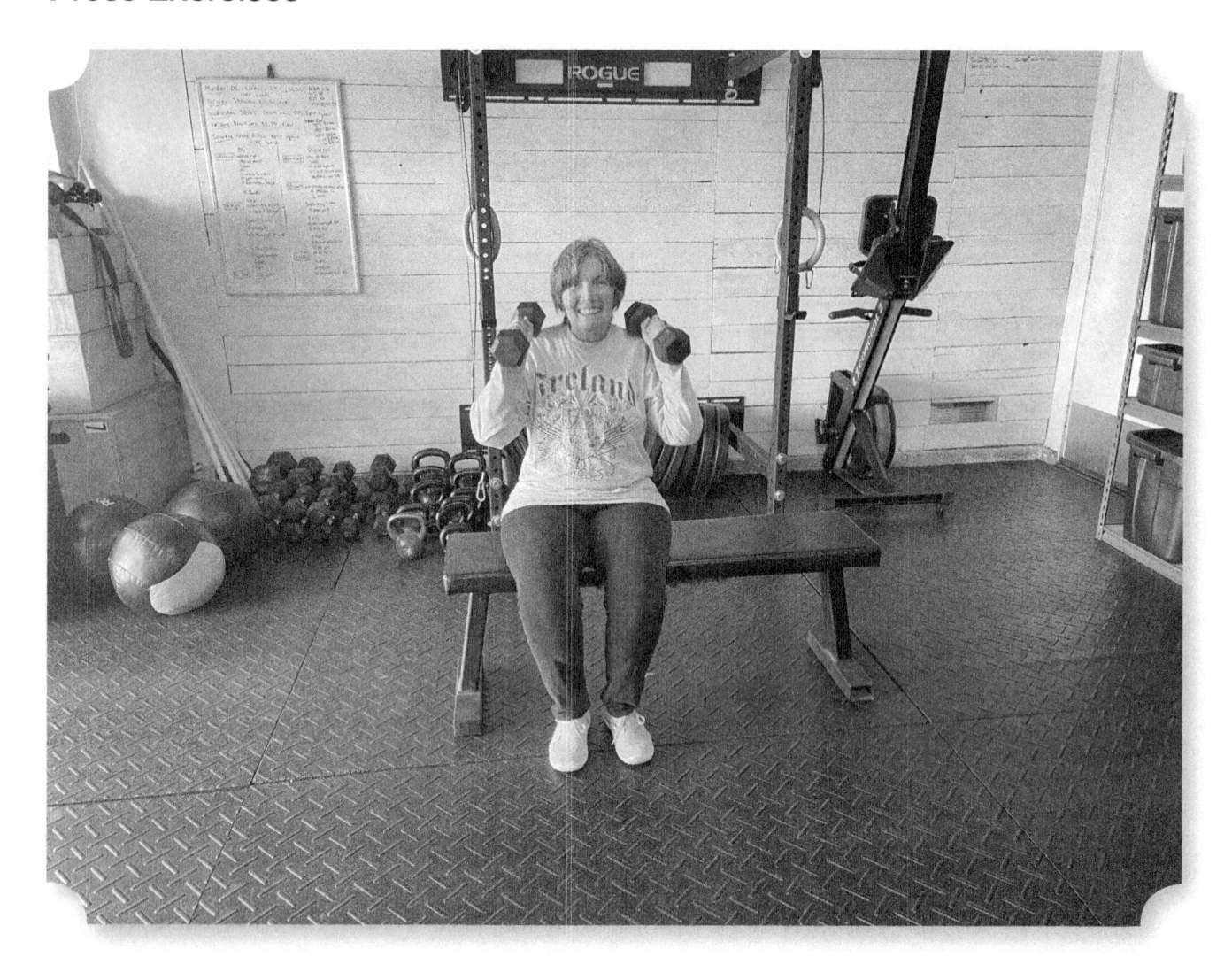

Shoulder Press

The shoulder press exercise can be done seated. Sit up as straight as you can, tighten your abs, and hold a dumbbell in each hand with your palms facing each other. The dumbbells should be at shoulder height or just higher than your shoulders. Press your arms overhead. Raise the dumbbells overhead until your arms are straight but not locked. Lower the dumbbells back down to shoulder level and repeat. Do three sets of 10 presses. Rest one minute between each set. This exercise, done with muscle control and not momentum, will build strength in your upper body.

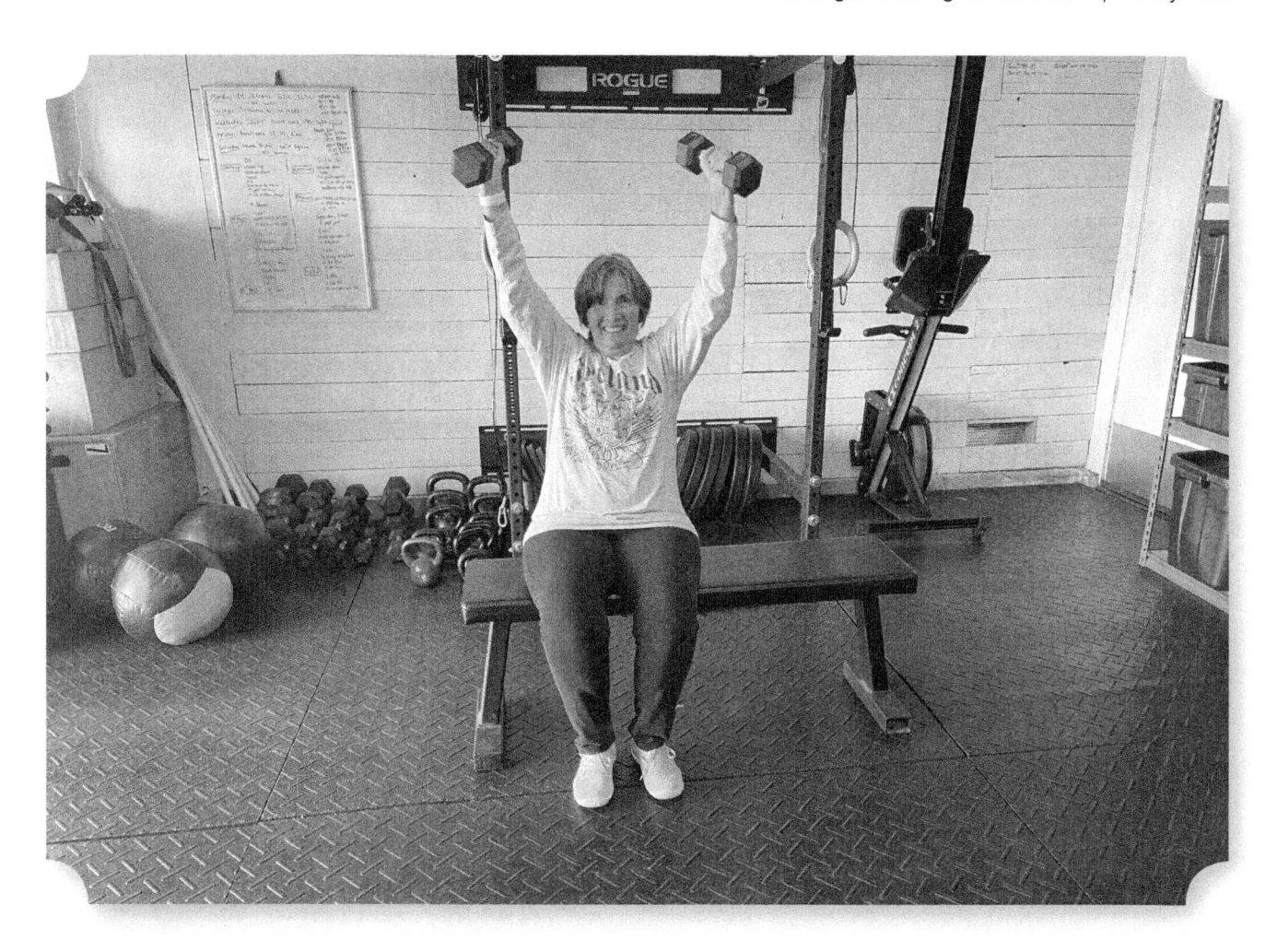

The bench press and seated anchored chest press are functional press exercises that can be added to your workout for variation.

Bench Press

A bench press needs sturdy support to lie down on and a bar to press up. To do a bench press, lie down on your back and hold the bar with both hands a little wider than shoulder-width apart. Press the bar up with both hands until your arms are straight but not locked, then lower it back down toward your chest. This exercise is also performed using muscle control instead of momentum. The bar doesn't need weights on it and even an ordinary broomstick will do. High repetitions of the movement will build strength in your torso, arms, and shoulders.

Seated Anchored Chest Press

Anchor the middle of a resistance band by looping it around a sturdy railing, bedpost, or another object at a height that is slightly higher than your shoulders. If you don't have such an object but have an exercise partner, your partner can hold the middle of the band. Sit facing away from your anchor and hold the ends of the band in each hand. Start the exercise with your hands just in front of your shoulders and press your hands forward until your arms are straight. Move your hands back to shoulder level and repeat the press 10 times. Do three sets with one minute rest between sets.

Variations for the Mobility-Impaired

For seniors who have limited mobility, the wall push-up can be a good alternative press exercise to maintain upper body strength and mobility. Stand facing a wall with your arms straight out in front of you and your palms flat against the wall. Slowly lean into the wall, bending your elbows and bringing your chest closer to the wall. Hold for a second, then slowly push back to the starting position.

Push Exercises

Your upper body has two basic movements: push and pull. These movements are subdivided into vertical and horizontal motions. When you create your exercise program, include functional opposites. For every pull, include a push. For every horizontal movement, include a vertical one.

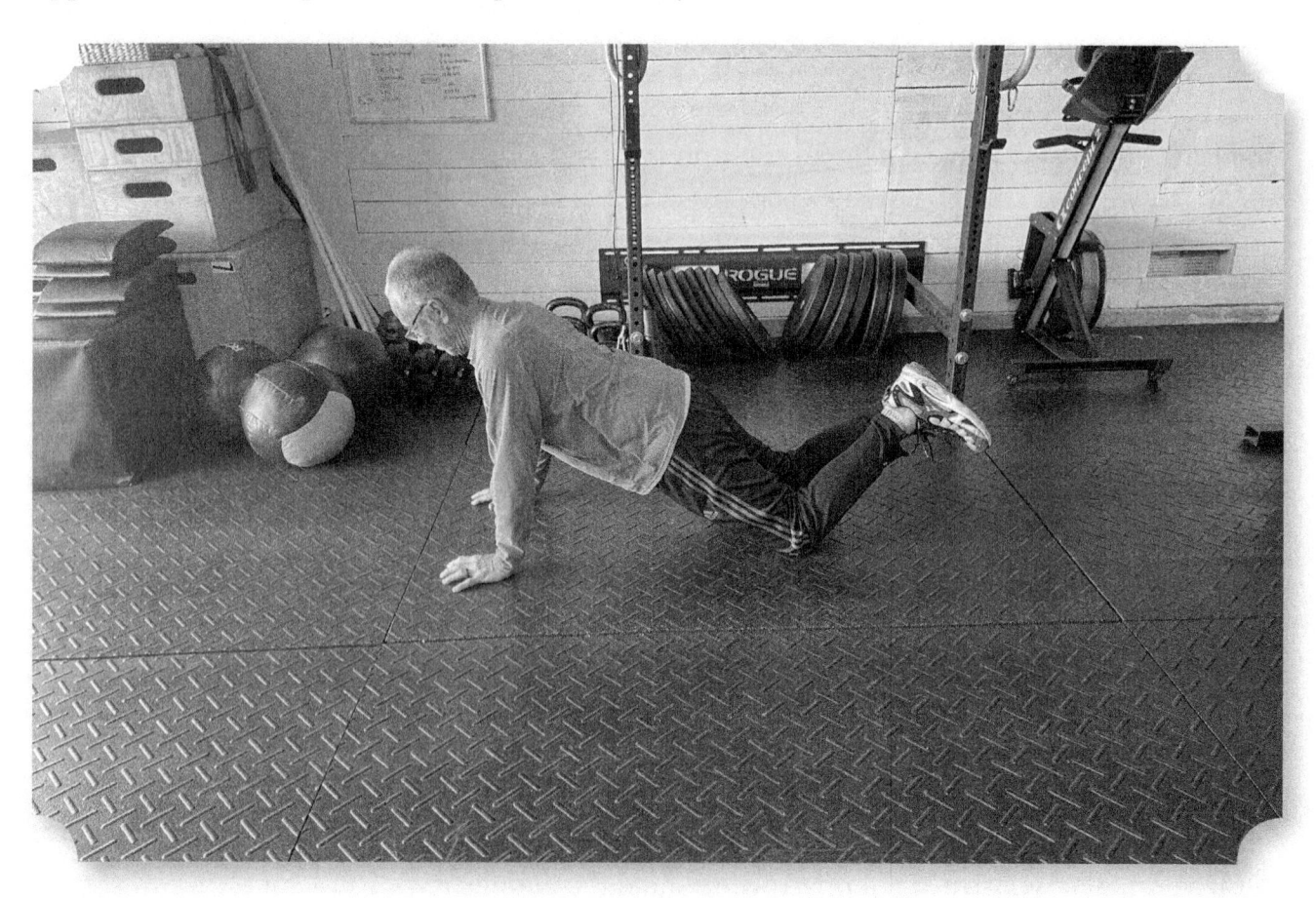

One of the most basic—and effective—push exercises is the common push-up. This exercise will strengthen your core, hips, glutes, and thighs. The push-up is simple: Push your upper body up until your arms are straight and lower yourself down in a controlled (not falling) movement. Don't arch your back and keep your hands just wider than shoulder-width. Keep your knees on the floor and aim for 10 repetitions. As your strength increases, you can increase the challenge to your muscles by gradually adding another set of 10 repetitions.

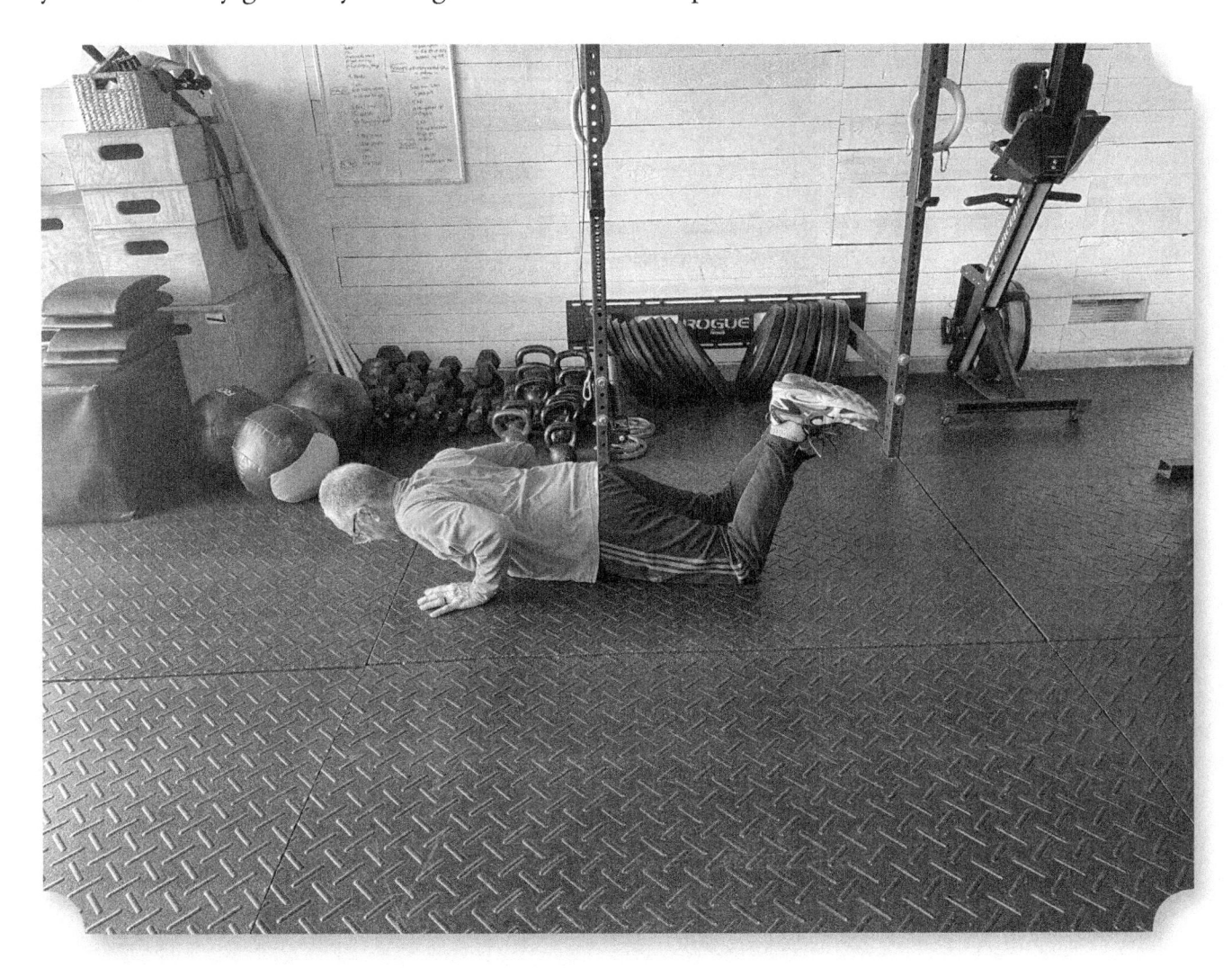

Variations for the Mobility-Impaired

If you are mobility-impaired, functional push exercises can help strengthen your upper body and improve your daily life activities. The seated chest press and the chest fly will improve strength in your upper body.

To do the seated chest press, sit on a sturdy chair with your back straight and your feet flat on the ground. Hold a pair of light dumbbells at chest height with your elbows bent and pointing out to the sides. Push the dumbbells away from your chest, straightening your arms, then bring them back to the starting position.

The chest fly is another push variation suitable for the mobility-impaired. Lie on your back on a mat or bed with your arms extended out to the sides and holding light dumbbells. Slowly bring your arms together above your chest, then lower them back to the starting position.

Pull Exercises

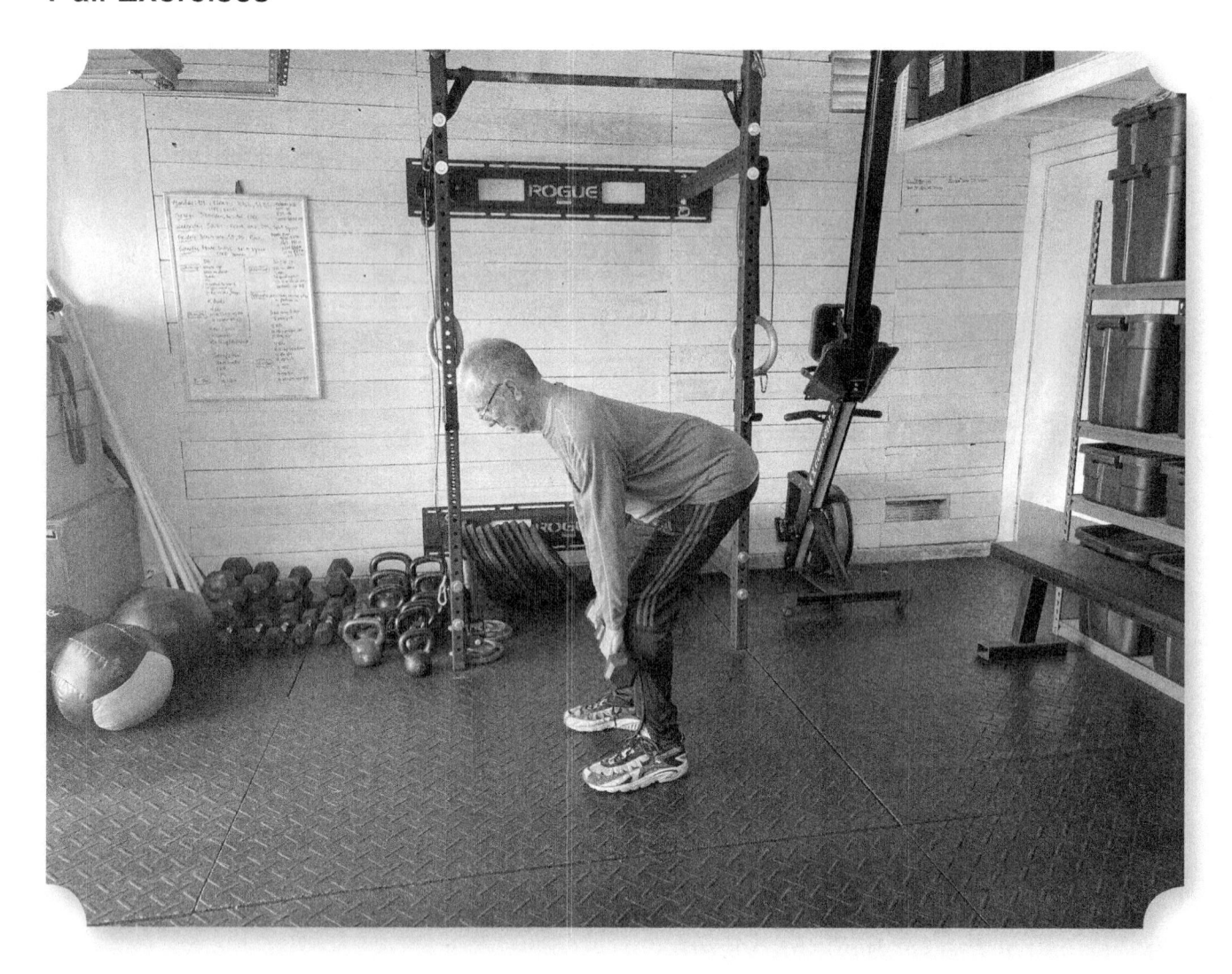

The resistance band pull will increase strength in the core, arms, and shoulders. This exercise can be done while standing or seated on the ground or on a chair. Start by looping a resistance band around the feet or hold a set of dumbbells with your palms facing your legs. Start in a squatting position. Tighten your abs and pull the band back or raise the dumbbells until you are standing up straight. Be aware of your posture to make sure you don't risk injury by arching your back or neck. Do 10 pulls. You can use resistance bands with various tension levels or dumbbells with various weights, depending on your ability. As your strength increases, you can gradually add more repetitions.

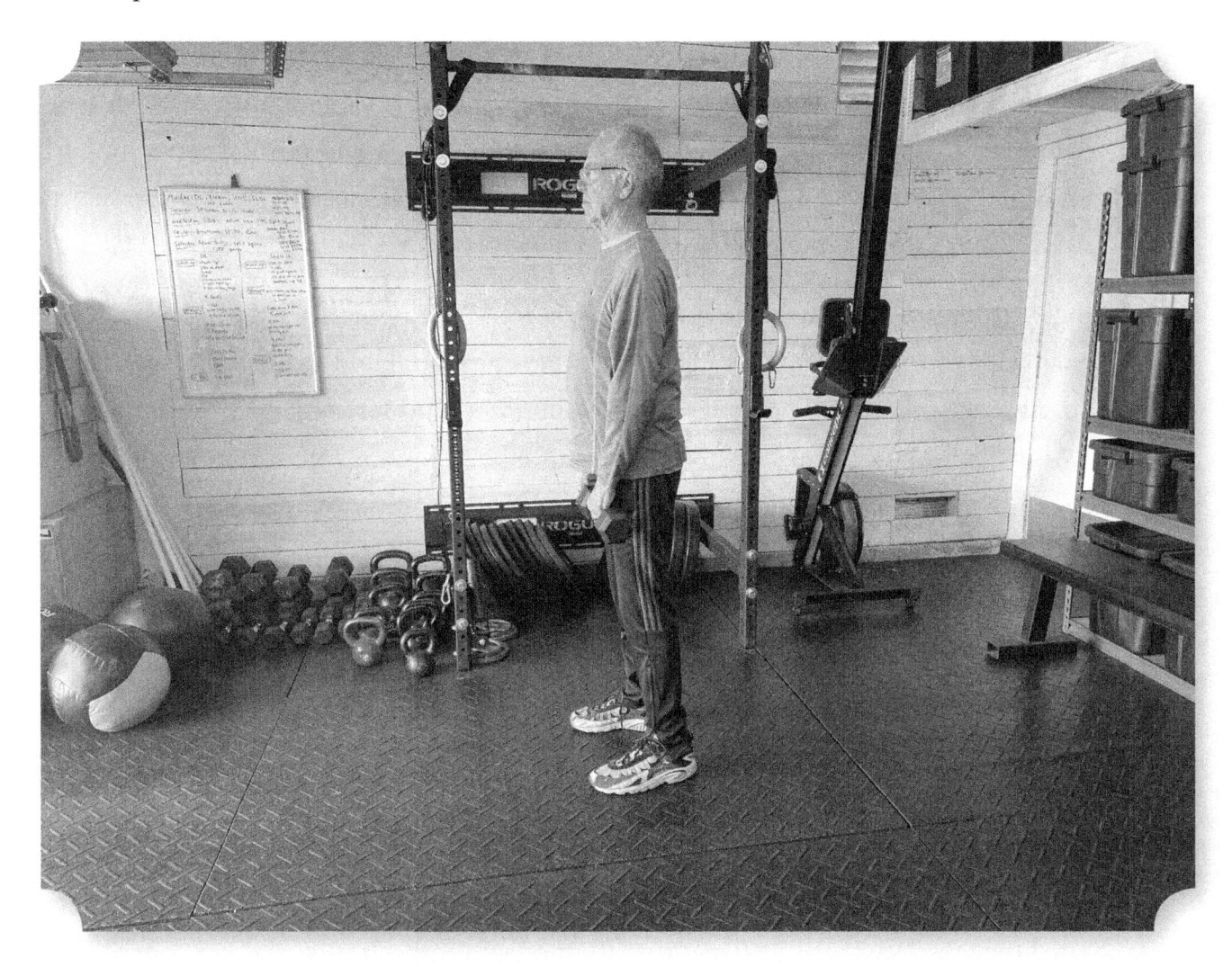

Variations for the Mobility-Impaired

If you find the standard pull exercises too difficult or you want to add variety to your workout, give these exercises a try:

- Seated row: This exercise targets the muscles in the upper back and arms. Sit on a bench with your feet flat on the ground. Attach a resistance band to a stable object and hold the other end with both hands. Pull the band toward your chest, keeping your elbows close to your body. Slowly release back to the starting position.

- Cable pull-down: This exercise targets the muscles in the shoulders and upper back. Sit in a chair with your feet flat on the ground and attach a resistance band to a stable object above your head. Hold the other end of the band with both hands and pull it down toward your chest, keeping your elbows close to your body. Slowly release back to the starting position.

- Door pulls: This exercise targets the muscles in the upper back and arms. Attach a resistance band to a closed door at chest height. Hold the other end of the band with both hands and pull it toward your chest, keeping your elbows close to your body. Slowly release back to the starting position.

- Single-arm rows: This exercise targets the muscles in the upper back and arms. Sit on a bench with your legs extended and feet flat on the ground. Hold a dumbbell in one hand and place the other hand on your thigh for support. Bend forward at the waist and pull the dumbbell toward your chest, keeping your elbow close to your body. Slowly release back to the starting position.

General Functional Exercises for the Mobility-Impaired

These exercises are not only for the mobility-impaired who might need variations on the regular exercises—they are for anyone who wants to change or add to their routine.

- Seated marching: While sitting in a chair, lift one knee up as high as possible and then lower it back down. Repeat with the other knee. This exercise can help strengthen the leg muscles and improve flexibility.

- Seated toe taps: While sitting in a chair, lift one foot off the ground and tap your toes on the floor in front of you. Then switch to the other foot. This exercise can help improve ankle mobility and circulation.

- Seated arm circles: While sitting in a chair, extend your arms out to your sides and make small circles with your hands. Repeat in the opposite direction. This exercise can help improve the range of motion in the shoulders.

- Seated leg extensions: While sitting in a chair, extend one leg straight out in front of you so that it is parallel to the ground and hold for a few seconds before lowering it back down. Repeat with the other leg. This exercise can help improve quad strength and flexibility.

- Seated shoulder rolls: While sitting in a chair, roll your shoulders forward and then backward in a circular motion. This exercise can help improve the range of motion in the shoulders and relieve tension in the neck and upper back.

- Seated heel raises: While sitting in a chair, keep your toes on the ground and lift your heels off the ground and then lower them back down. This exercise can help improve ankle mobility and calf strength.

Chapter 6:
Accessory Movements

Accessory movements are just as important as the functional movements discussed in Chapter 5. These movements are unilateral, meaning that you will use each arm or leg individually. Accessory movements work each muscle individually and with purpose.

Single-Leg Deadlift

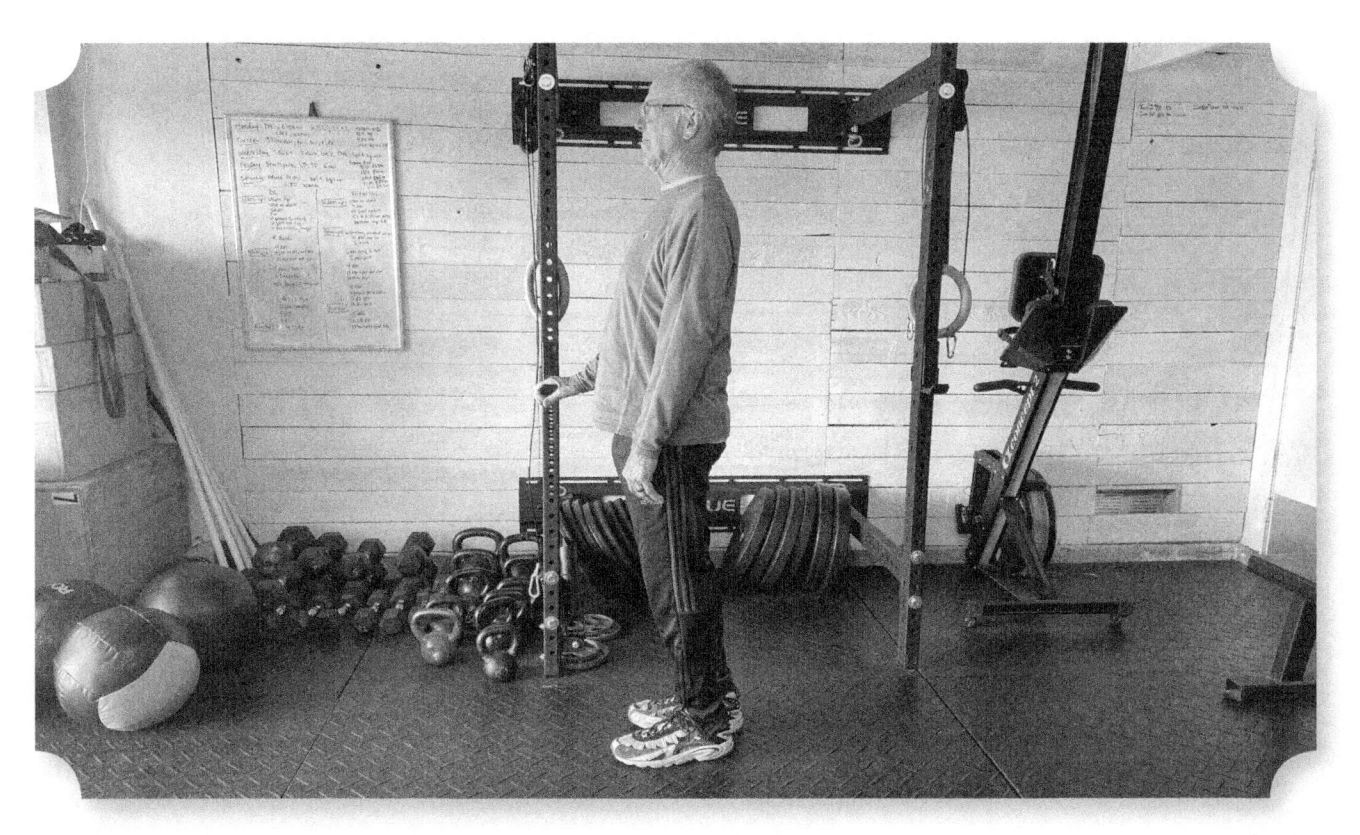

This exercise strengthens the muscles of the posterior chain. The posterior chain consists of the muscles of the lower back, glutes, hamstrings, and core. To do the single-leg deadlift, start by standing with your feet hip-width apart. Hold your right leg straight, but don't lock it. Move your left foot back as if you want to kick something behind you with your heel. Keep your left leg straight and hinge from the hip to lower your upper body until it is nearly parallel to the floor. During the exercise, keep your arms straight and perpendicular to the floor. The aim is to have your body in a straight line from your left foot to your head. Hinge back and return your straight left leg to the standing position. Repeat the movement with your left leg on the floor. If you are a beginner, do three sets of 10 repetitions for each leg. Rest for 90 seconds between each set. As your balance improves and the exercise starts to feel easy, do the single-leg deadlift with dumbbells.

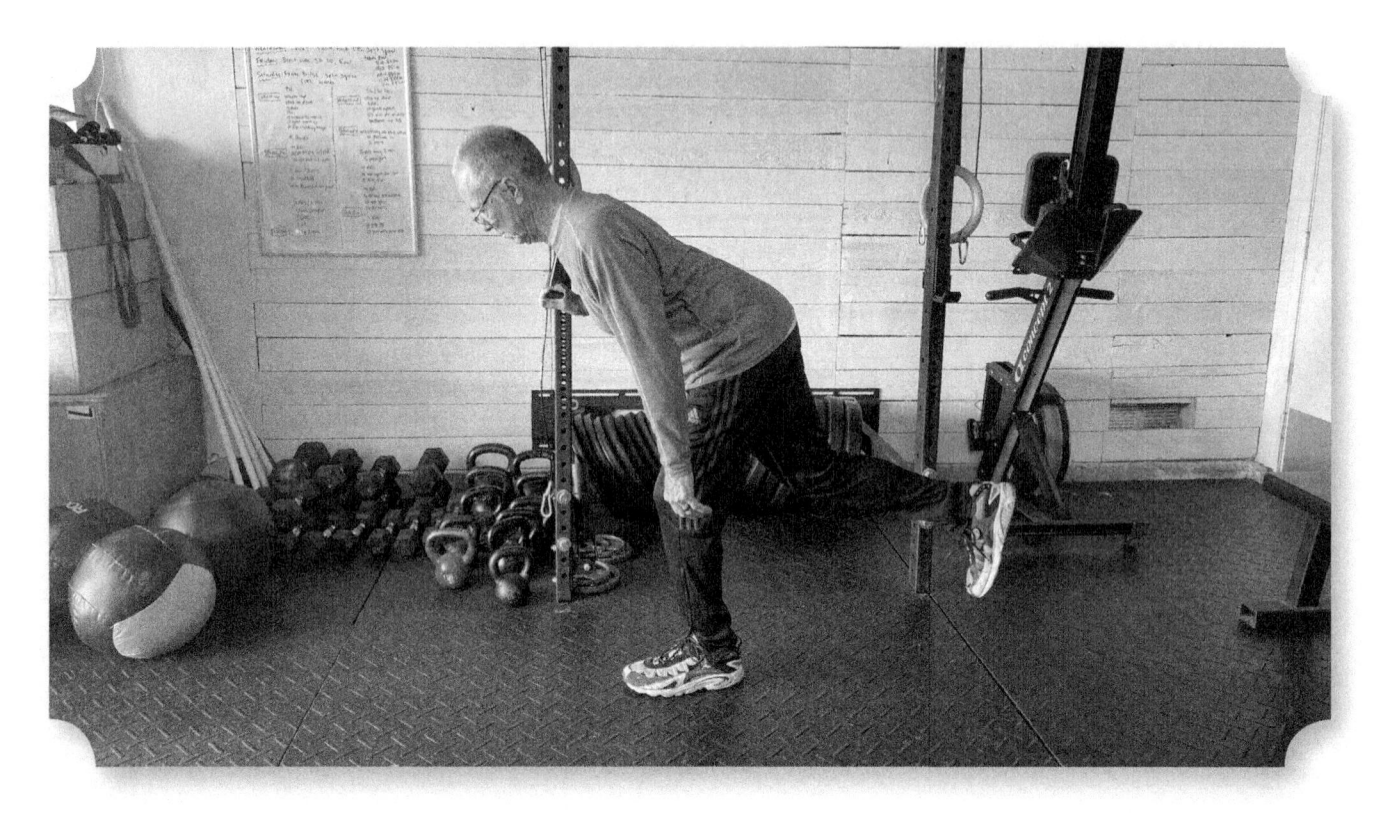

Variations for the Mobility-Impaired

Single-leg deadlifts can be a challenging exercise for seniors who have mobility impairments. However, there are several variations that can make this exercise more accessible and safer. Here are a few suggestions:

- Assisted single-leg deadlift: Use a sturdy chair or a wall to assist with balance. Stand facing the chair or wall with your feet hip-width apart. Shift your weight onto one leg and lift the other leg off the ground. Slowly hinge forward at the hips, reaching your opposite arm toward the chair or wall for support. Keep your back straight and your lifted leg straight as you lower your torso toward the ground. Pause at the bottom, then use your supporting leg to return to standing. Repeat on the other side.

- Single-leg deadlift with toe touch: Stand with your feet hip-width apart and lift one leg off the ground. Slowly hinge forward at the hips, reaching your opposite hand toward your lifted foot. Keep your back straight and your lifted leg straight as you lower your torso toward the ground. Pause at the bottom, then use your supporting leg to return to standing. Repeat on the other side.

- Single-leg deadlift with band assistance: Attach a resistance band to a sturdy anchor point, such as a doorknob or post. Hold onto the band with both hands and step into it with one foot. Shift your weight onto the banded foot and lift the other foot off the ground. Slowly hinge forward at the hips, using the band for support as you lower your torso toward the ground and keep your back straight and your lifted leg straight. Pause at the bottom, then use your supporting leg to return to standing. Repeat on the other side.

Single-Arm Bent-Over Row

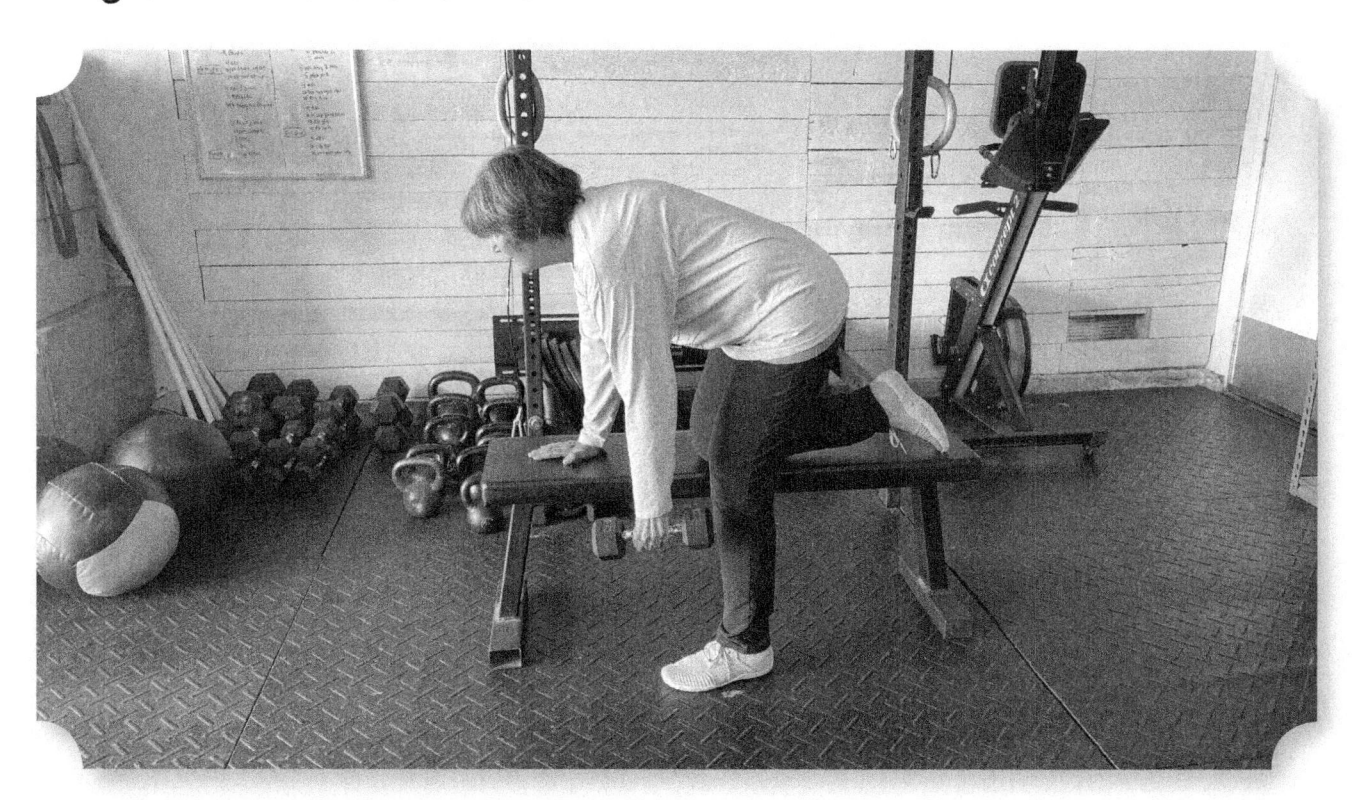

This exercise strengthens the back muscles. Start by standing up straight next to your bench, box, or chair with the dumbbell resting on the floor. Put your left knee on your bench and pick the dumbbell up with your right hand. Your right arm should be straight and your left hand resting on the bench. To avoid the risk of injury, don't bend your neck to look up toward the ceiling. Tuck your right elbow close to your side and pull the dumbbell toward your chest until it touches the side of your chest. Lower the dumbbell back to the starting position by using a slow, controlled movement. When doing this exercise, be careful to not round your back or twist your upper body when you pull the dumbbell up. Do three sets of 10 rows for each arm, and rest for 90 seconds between each set.

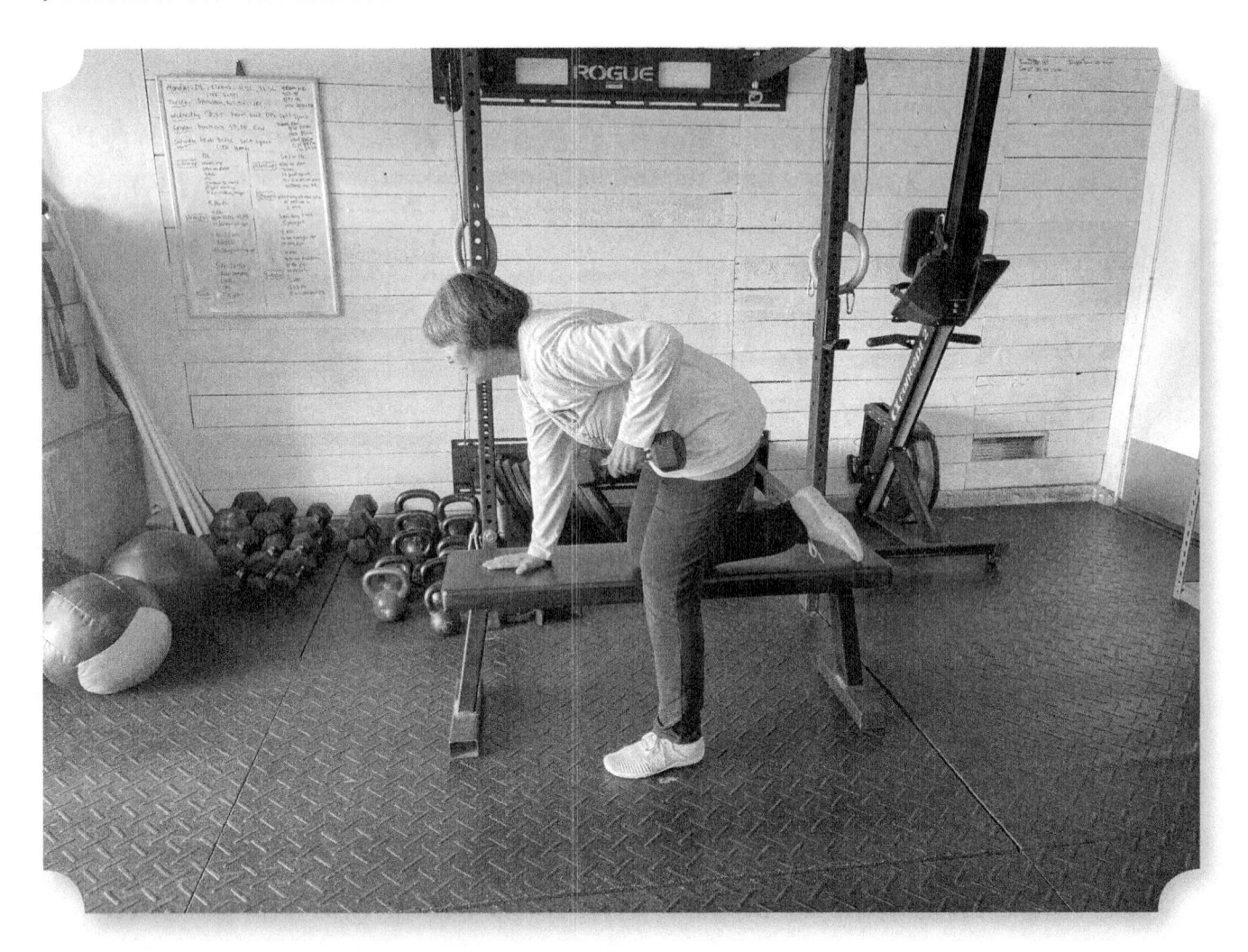

Variations for the Mobility-Impaired

The single-arm bent-over row is a great exercise for building upper body strength, but depending on your level of mobility, modifications may be necessary. Here are some variations of the single-arm bent-over row that are suitable for the needs of seniors with mobility limitations:

- Seated single-arm row: This variation can be done in a chair or wheelchair. Sit with your feet flat on the floor and grasp a dumbbell or resistance band with one hand. Hold the dumbbell on your thigh, palm facing downward. If you are working with a resistance band, you can loop the band around your foot. Bend your elbow, pulling the weight up toward your chest, keeping your elbow close to your body, then lower the weight back down to your thigh.

- Standing single-arm row with support: Stand facing a wall or sturdy piece of furniture with your feet shoulder-width apart. Hold onto the support with one hand and grasp a dumbbell or resistance band in your other hand. Bend your elbow, pulling the weight up toward your chest, keeping your elbow close to your body, then lower the weight back down to the starting position to complete one repetition.

- Seated cable single-arm row: This variation requires access to a cable machine but can be done while seated, making it a good option for seniors with limited mobility. Sit facing the cable machine with your feet flat on the floor. Grasp the handle with one hand and row the cable toward your chest, keeping your elbow close to your body. Lower the weight back down to complete one repetition.

- Seated single-arm row with no weight: This variation is a good starting point for seniors who are new to strength training or have limited mobility. Sit with your feet flat on the floor and place your hand on your knee. Engage your back muscles and pull your elbow back toward your hip, squeezing your shoulder blade. Lower your arm back down. As you get stronger, you can progress to the seated single-arm row.

Reverse Lunge

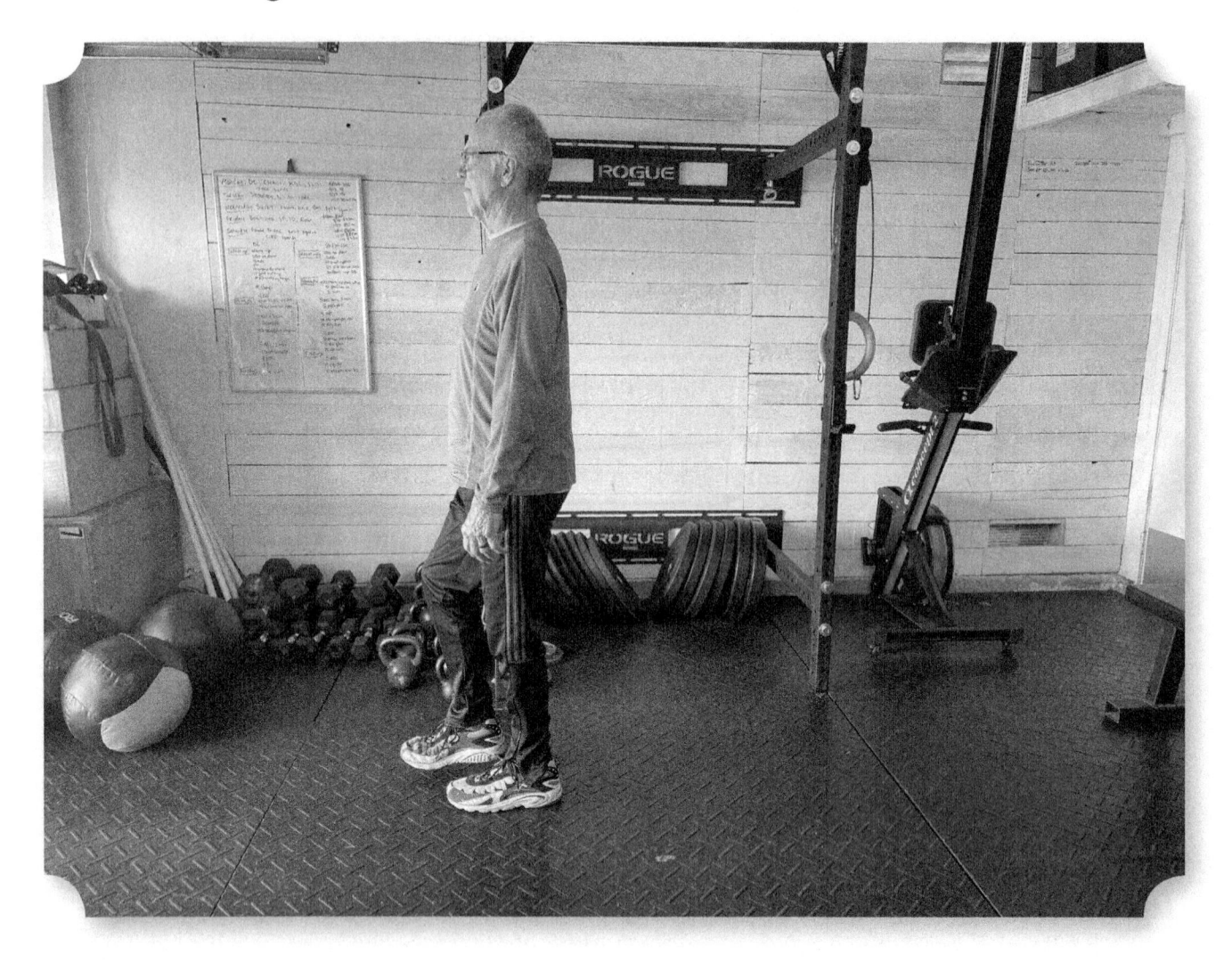

The reverse lunge will build strength in your legs and improve your balance. To start, stand up as straight as you can with your feet shoulder-width apart. If you are a beginner, don't hold any weights in your hands until you can easily do 10 lunges for each leg. You can gradually add weights as you get stronger. If you are already strong enough to do so, and you don't have balance issues, you can hold a dumbbell or a kettlebell in each hand. While lowering your hips toward the floor, lunge backward with your right leg. Avoid injury by being careful to not move your leg back past your comfort zone. When you have reached the bottom of your lunge, push yourself up with both your legs. Repeat the movements with your left leg lunging backward. A set will be 10 lunges with each leg. Do three sets with a 90-second rest in between.

Keeping the correct form will guard you against injury and ensure that you reap the full benefits of the reverse lunge. At the bottom of the lunge, your front thigh should be parallel to the ground. Don't lift the heel of the front foot during the lunge. Hold your back straight and keep your head neutral by looking forward and not raising or dropping your chin. When you are lowering yourself, inhale deeply. Exhale while pushing yourself up. Keep the middle of your front knee in line with your middle toe. Tighten your core throughout the entire exercise.

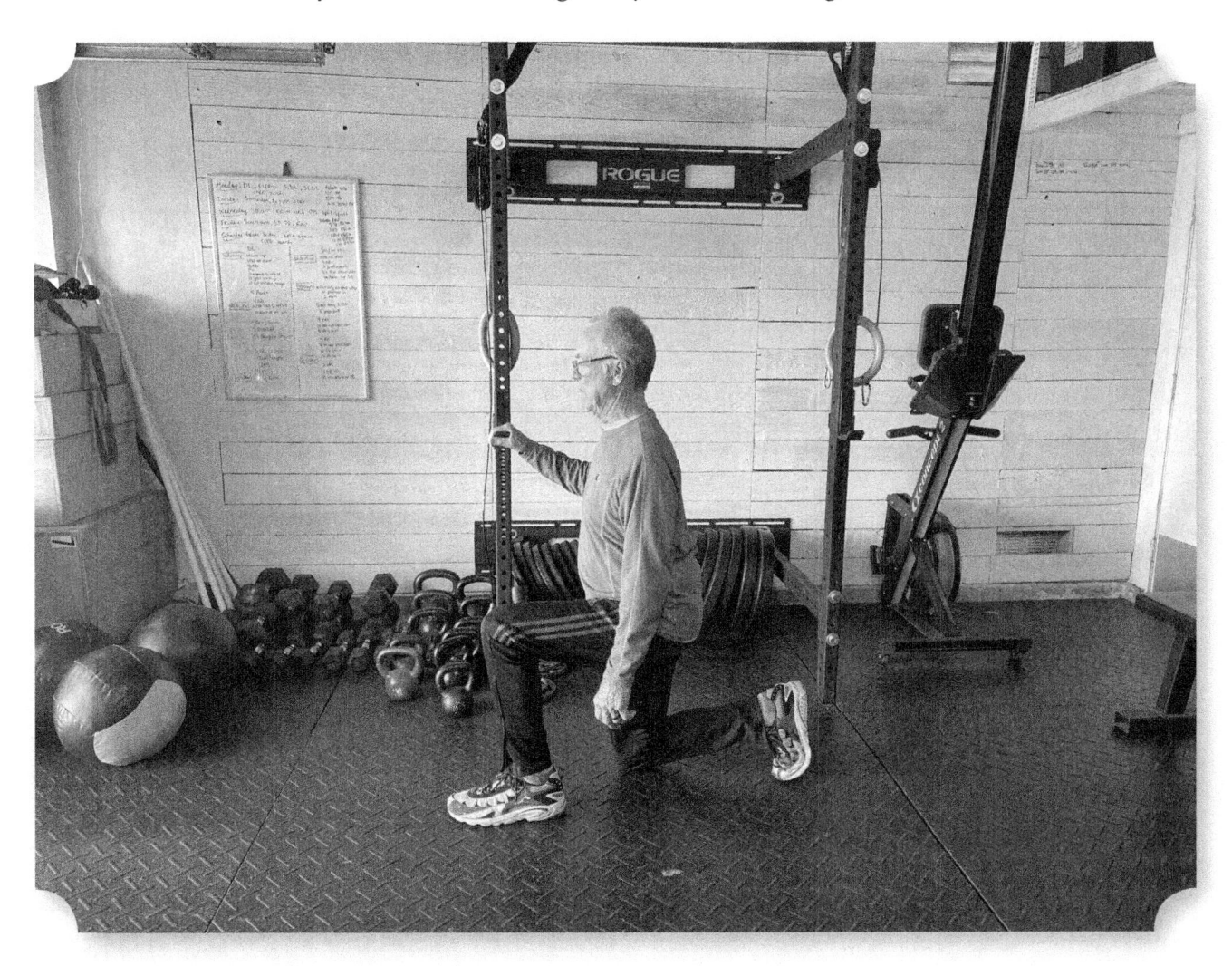

Variations for the Mobility-Impaired

Reverse lunges can be a great exercise for improving lower body strength and mobility, but for those who may have limited mobility or balance issues, several variations can be done to make the exercise more accessible.

- Lunge with chair support: Stand facing a chair with your hands resting on the back of it. Step back with one foot and lower your body until your back knee almost touches the ground. Return to the starting position and repeat with the other leg.

- Stationary lunges: Instead of stepping back and forth, simply lunge down and up on the spot. This can help with balance and stability as you are not shifting your weight as much.

- Wall-assisted lunges: Stand facing a wall with your hands resting on it for support. Step back with one foot and lower your body until your back knee almost touches the ground. Move back up until your legs are straight but not locked, and repeat with the other leg.

Split Squat

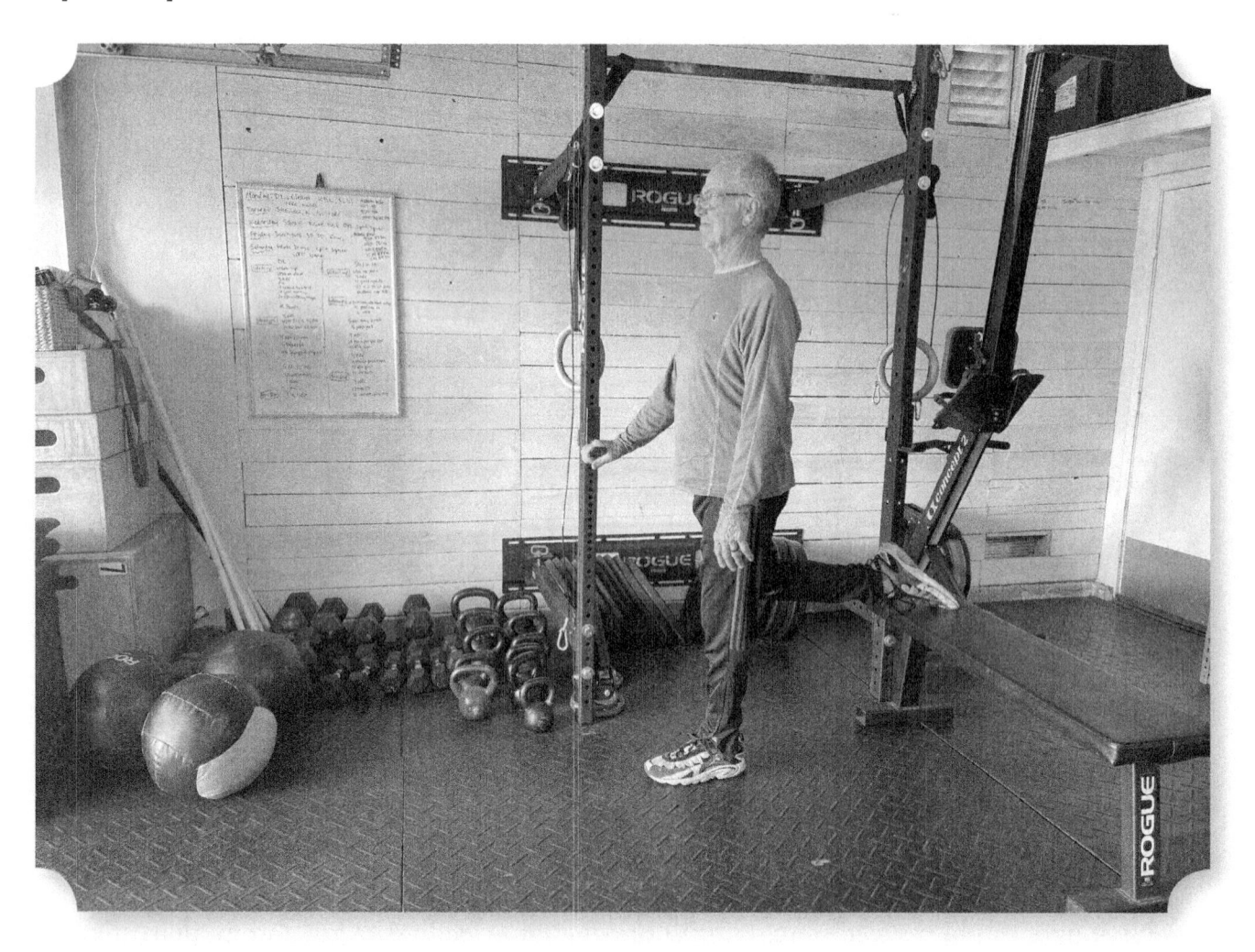

An ordinary squat will strengthen the leg muscles. By doing single-leg squats, you add the benefit of a highly efficient balance training exercise. Another bonus is that the split squat doesn't put any load on your lower back, and because you can lower yourself further than with an ordinary squat, your hips will develop more flexibility. Your foot position will determine which muscle groups are the most targeted. The further your front foot is from the elevated surface, the more your glutes and hamstrings will be worked. Putting your front foot closer to the elevated surface will result in your quadriceps—the muscles in the front of your thighs—getting most of the workout. If you choose a closer position, don't let your front knee go further forward than your toes. Experiment with what feels the most comfortable and natural for you.

You will need a sturdy, nonslip knee-high surface such as a bench, box, or chair. Stand in front of the bench, feet shoulder-width apart, and take a step forward. Stand on your left leg and put the foot of your right leg on the bench. Tighten your core and lean slightly forward at the waist, not the shoulders. Bend your left leg and lower yourself down slowly. If your front foot is further from the bench, the bottom of your movement is when your thigh is parallel to the floor. If your foot is in a closer position and you feel the stretch more in your glutes than quadriceps (quads), then the bottom of the squat is just before your knee would be over your toes. After reaching the bottom of your squat, push yourself up by driving through your front foot using your leg muscles.

If you are a beginner, start with two sets of eight repetitions with each leg. Rest 90 seconds between each set. Gradually add a repetition until you can easily do three sets of 12. At that level, you can hold a dumbbell in each hand to keep the exercise challenging for your muscles.

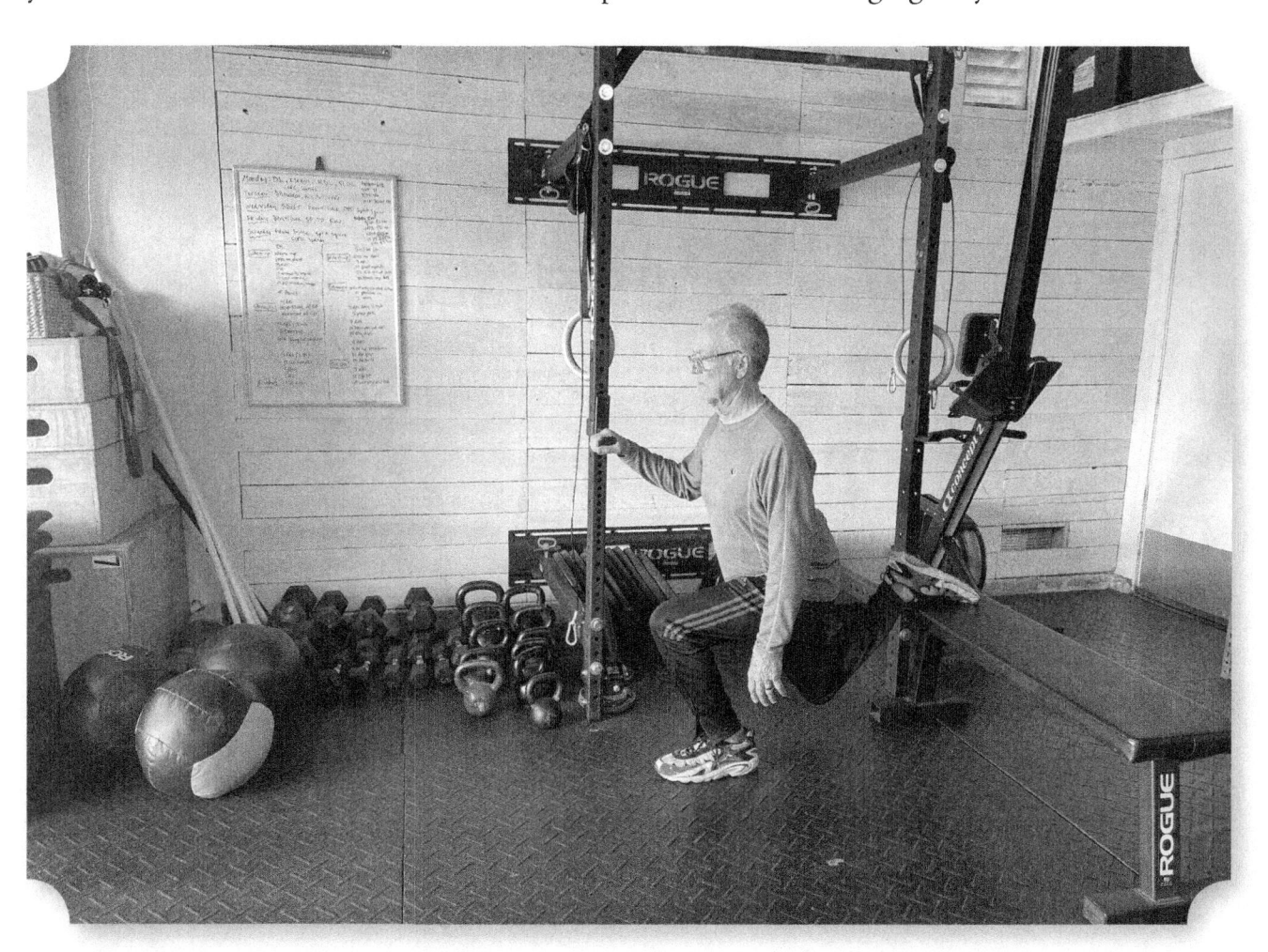

Variations for the Mobility-Impaired

If you are mobility-impaired, it may be difficult to perform a traditional split squat. However, several variations can be used to make the exercise more accessible. Here are some suggestions:

- Wall-supported split squat: Stand facing a wall and place your hands on it for support. Step one foot back into a lunge position with your front knee directly above your ankle. Return to the standing position and repeat with your other leg.

- Chair-supported split squat: Place a chair or stable object in front of you and hold onto it for support. Step one foot back into a lunge position and lower your back knee toward the ground. Push through your front heel to stand up and repeat on the other side.

- Split squat with elevated front foot: Stand with one foot on an elevated surface, such as a step or box. Step the other foot back into a lunge position and lower your back knee toward the ground. Stand up and repeat the lunge with your other leg.

- Split squat with isometric hold: Stand with your feet hip-width apart and step one foot back into a lunge position. Lower your back knee toward the ground and hold the position for five seconds before standing up and repeating on the other side.

Thruster

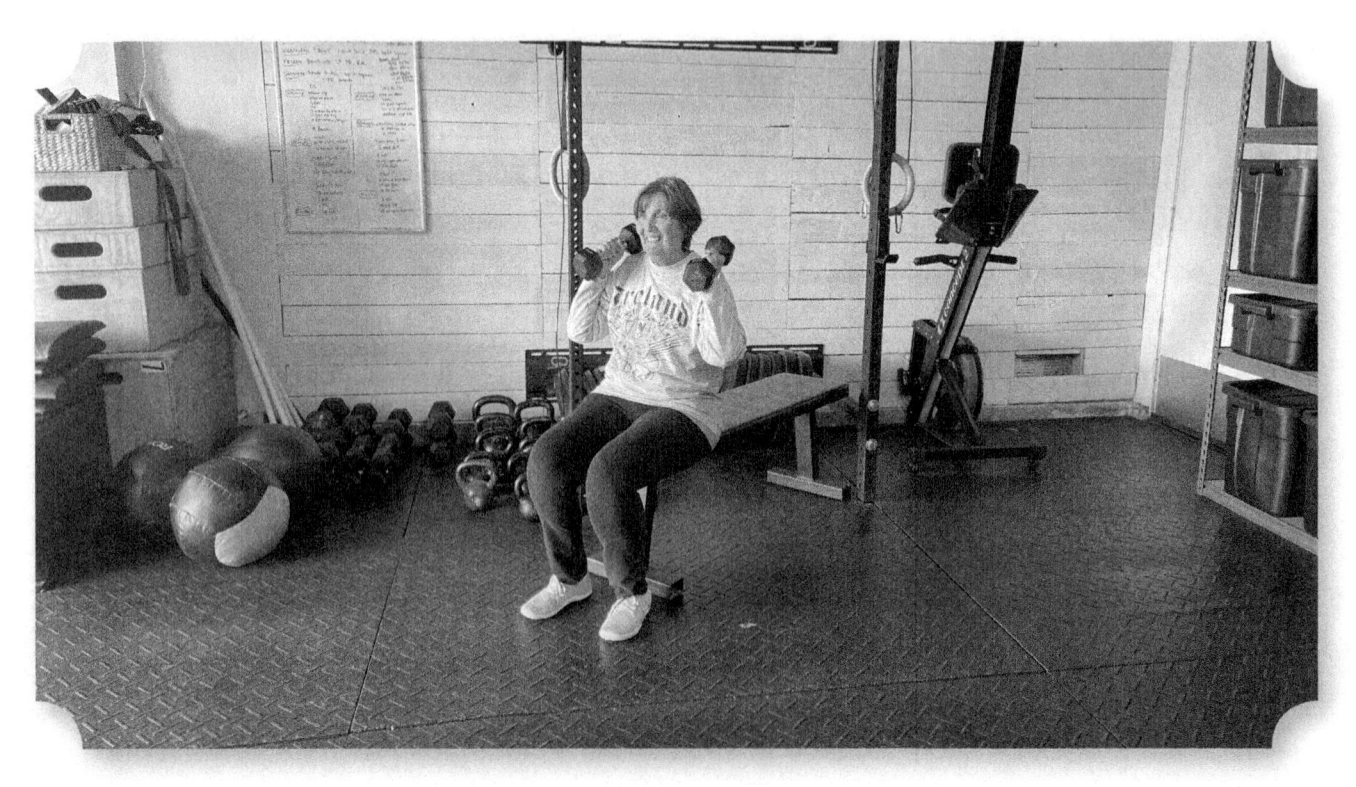

This exercise is a combination of the squat-to-chair and the overhead press. The thruster uses the entire body to improve your core, upper body, and lower body. Doing thrusters consistently will improve your balance and stamina as well. To reduce any risk of injury, use only smooth and controlled movements. Don't be tempted to use momentum or break the exercise up into a series of smaller movements.

Start out sitting on a bench and holding a dumbbell in each hand with your feet shoulder-width apart. If you are a beginner, do thrusters without any weights until you are used to the movements. Hold the dumbbells slightly higher than your shoulders with your palms facing your head. Keep an eye on your posture and make sure your shoulders are down and back and that your back is straight throughout this exercise. Tighten your core and stand up while raising the dumbbells overhead until your arms are straight but not locked. Lower the dumbbells down to your shoulders as you sit back down. Use your muscles in a controlled manner. If you are a beginner, set a goal to complete 10 repetitions. As your muscles gain strength, you can gradually add more sets to your workout.

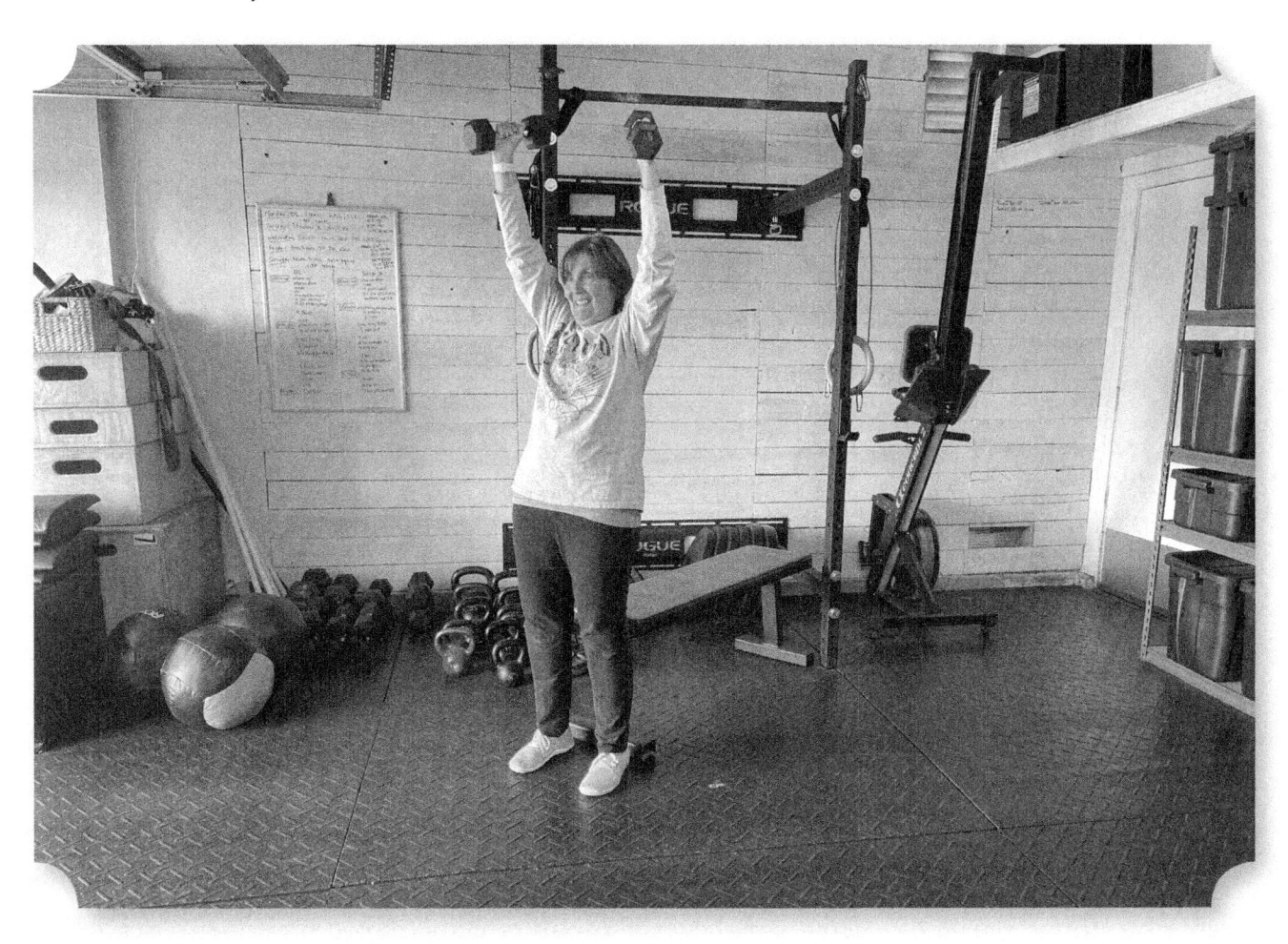

Variations for the Mobility-Impaired

If you find it too difficult to do the squat part of the exercise, step up onto a low sturdy box or stair with one or both feet and press the weight overhead, then step down and repeat on the other side.

Chest Press on the Ground With Dumbbells

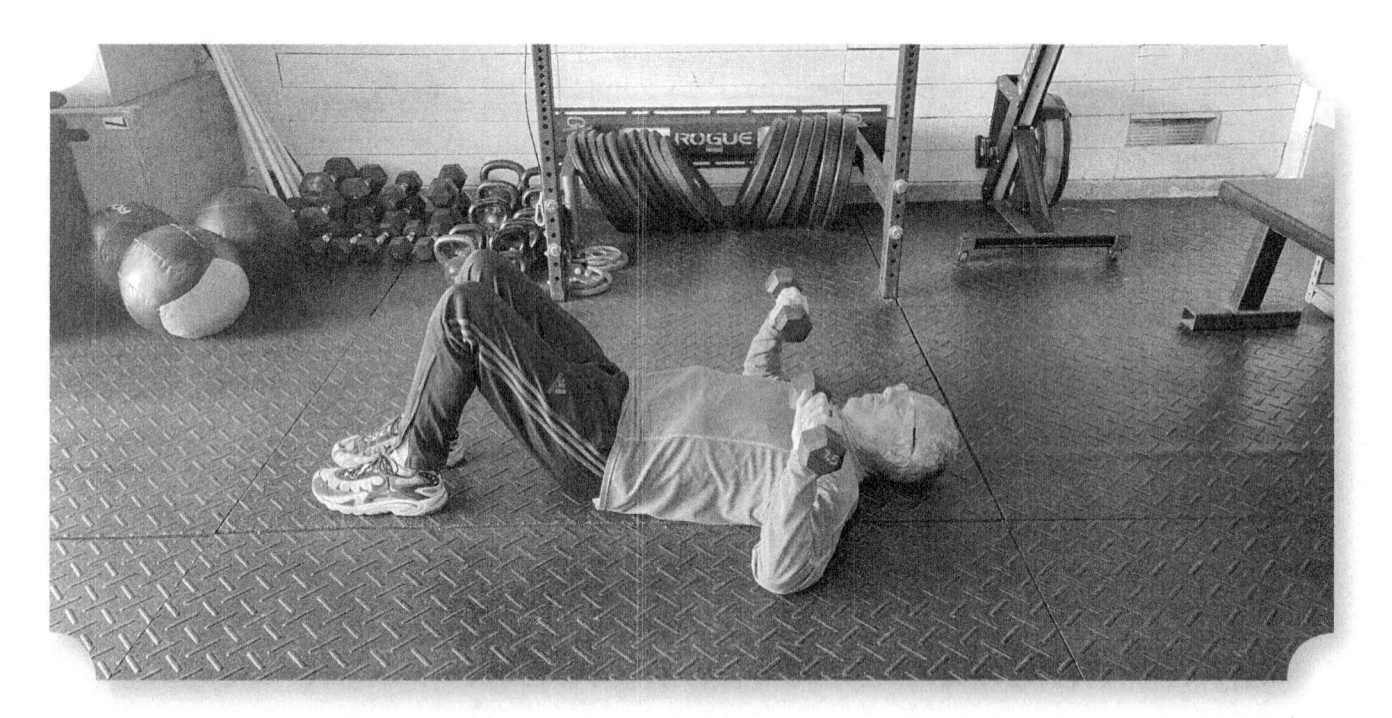

The chest press is a common strength training exercise that targets the chest muscles, shoulders, and triceps. This is a modified version of the exercise done from the floor to reduce the risk of injury. To start, lie on your back on a comfortable, padded surface, such as a yoga mat, with your feet flat on the floor and your knees bent. Hold a pair of light dumbbells (start with 1–2 pounds) with your palms facing forward and your arms extended straight up toward the ceiling over your chest. Slowly lower the weights toward your chest, bending your elbows and keeping them close to your body. Pause when the weights are just above your chest and then slowly press them back up toward the ceiling, fully extending your arms. Repeat for 10–15 repetitions or as many as you can comfortably manage, focusing on slow, controlled movements. Choose weights that are appropriate for your fitness level and start with a lighter weight than you think you can handle. You can increase the weight as you get stronger and more familiar with the movements. Keep your movements slow and controlled to avoid injury and engage your muscles fully. Be mindful of your breathing, inhaling as you lower the weights and exhaling as you press them back up.

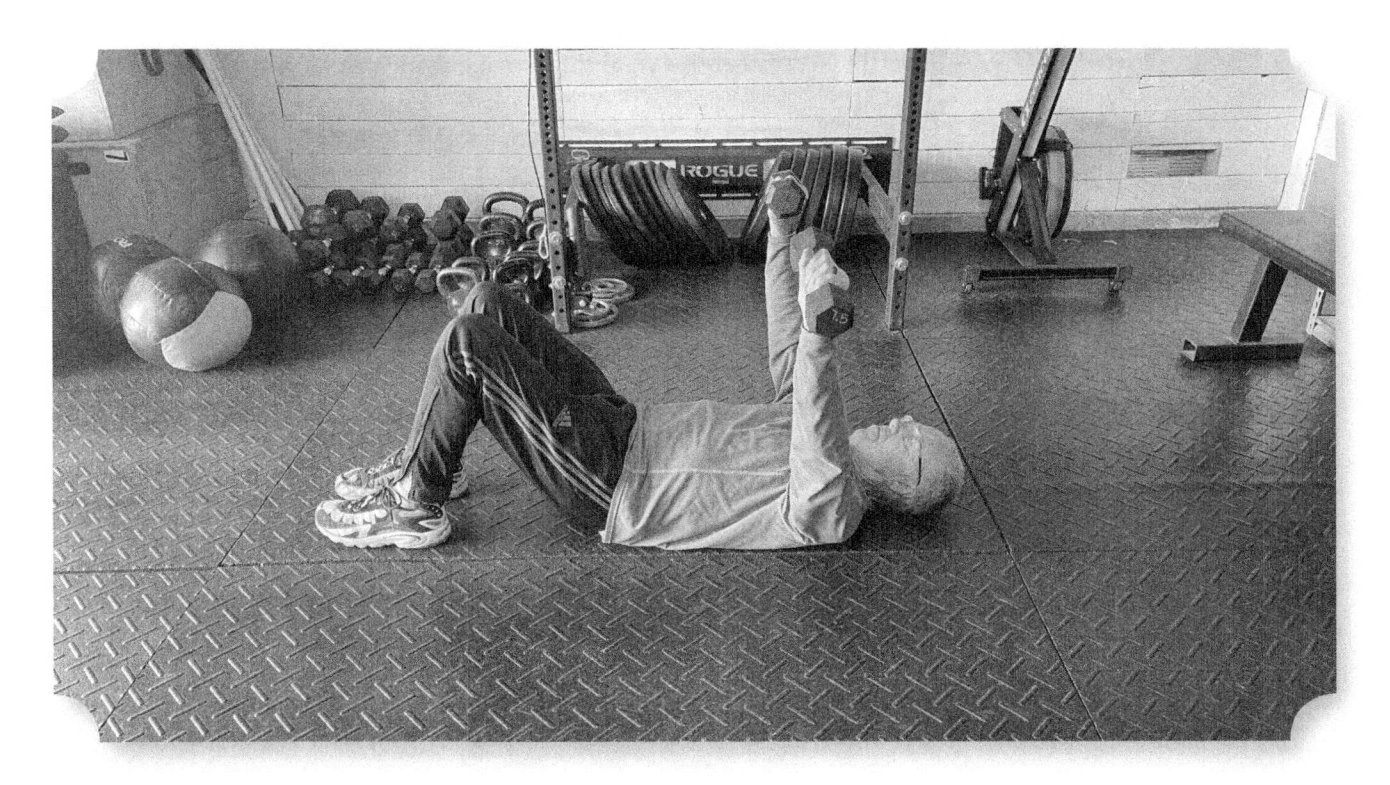

Variations for the Mobility-Impaired

If you have mobility impairments that limit your ability to perform traditional chest press exercises, there are several variations you can try:

- Seated chest press: If you have limited mobility in your legs or hips, you can perform a chest press while seated on a bench or chair. This will help you to stabilize your torso and focus on engaging your chest muscles.

- Incline chest press: If you have limited mobility in your shoulders or upper back, an incline chest press may be a good option. This involves performing a chest press on a bench that is angled at around 45 degrees, which can help to take some of the pressure off your shoulders.

- Resistance band chest press: If you have limited mobility in your wrists or hands, you can try using resistance bands instead of dumbbells. This will allow you to perform a chest press movement while holding onto the resistance bands with your palms facing inward.

- Machine chest press: If you have limited mobility in your upper body, you can try using a machine chest press. This type of exercise equipment will guide your movements and help you perform a chest press safely and effectively.

- Wall push-ups: If you have limited mobility in your arms, shoulders, or wrists, you can try doing wall push-ups. Stand facing a wall and place your hands on it at shoulder height. Slowly bend your arms, bringing your chest toward the wall, and then push yourself back up.

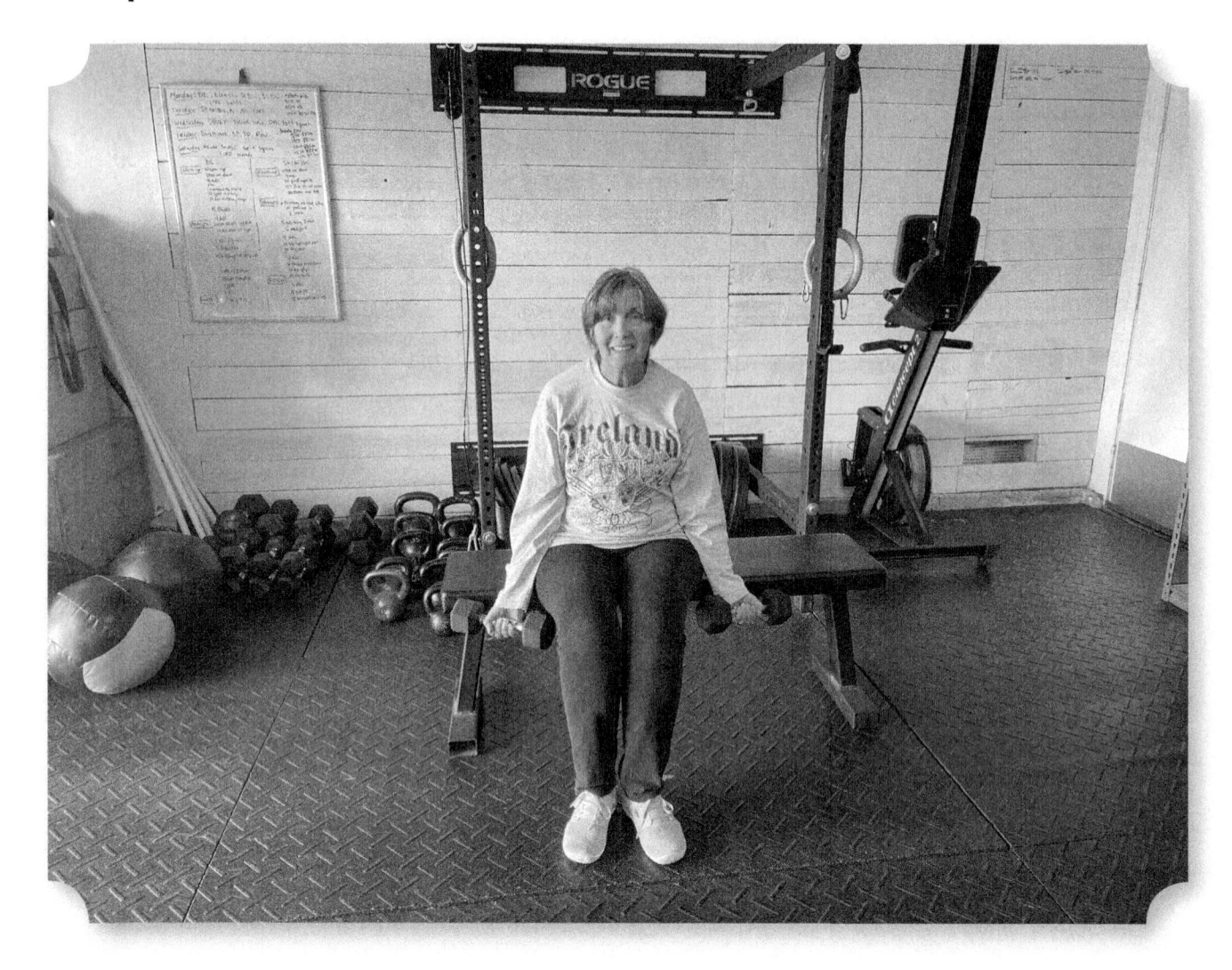

Bicep Curls

Bicep curls are a great exercise to build strength in the upper arm muscles, and they are easy to do. Start with light weights and gradually increase the weight as your strength improves. Stand or sit up straight with your feet shoulder-width apart. Keep your shoulders relaxed and down, and avoid hunching or arching your back. Slowly lift the weight toward your chest, keeping your elbows close to your body. Hold for a second, then lower the weight back down in a controlled manner. Exhale as you lift the weight, and inhale as you lower it. Aim for 10–15 repetitions and do 2–3 sets. Take a 2-minute break between sets.

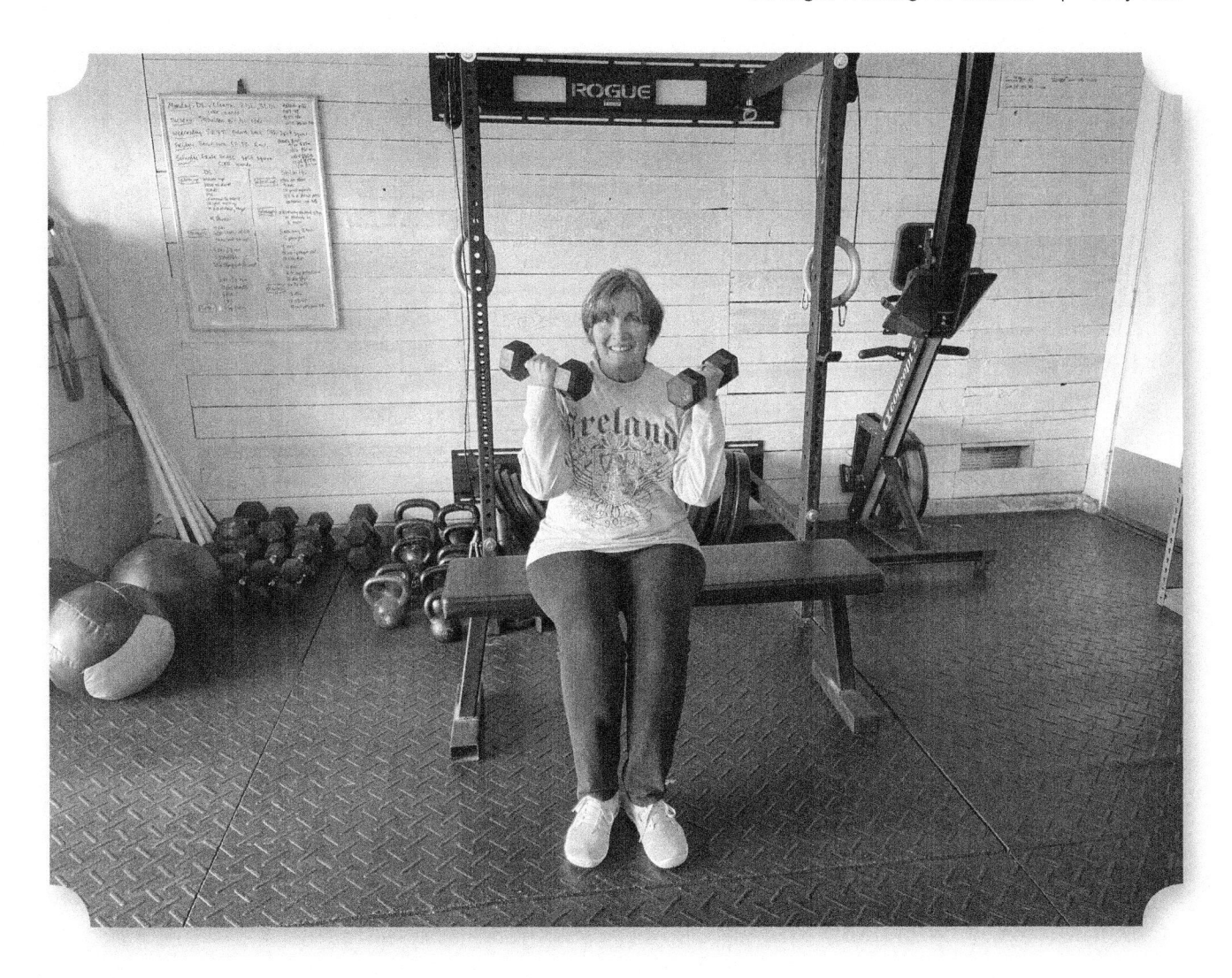

Variations for the Mobility-Impaired

If you have limited mobility in your upper body or arms, traditional bicep curls may be difficult or uncomfortable to perform. However, there are several variations of bicep curls that can be used to accommodate a wide range of mobility limitations. Here are some examples:

- Hammer curls: This variation of the bicep curl is performed with the palms facing each other rather than facing up. Hold a weight in each hand with your palms facing each other and your arms extended down by your sides. Curl the weights toward your shoulders, keeping your palms facing each other throughout the movement.

- Resistance band curls: If you have wrist problems that make it difficult to hold dumbbells, resistance bands are a great alternative. Secure the band under your feet and hold the other end in each hand. Curl the band toward your shoulders, keeping your elbows close to your sides.

- Isometric bicep curls: This variation involves holding a dumbbell in your hand and lifting it slightly but not moving it all the way to your shoulder. Hold the dumbbell in this position for a few seconds before lowering it back down. This movement can be done with or without a dumbbell and can be performed seated or standing.

Box Dips

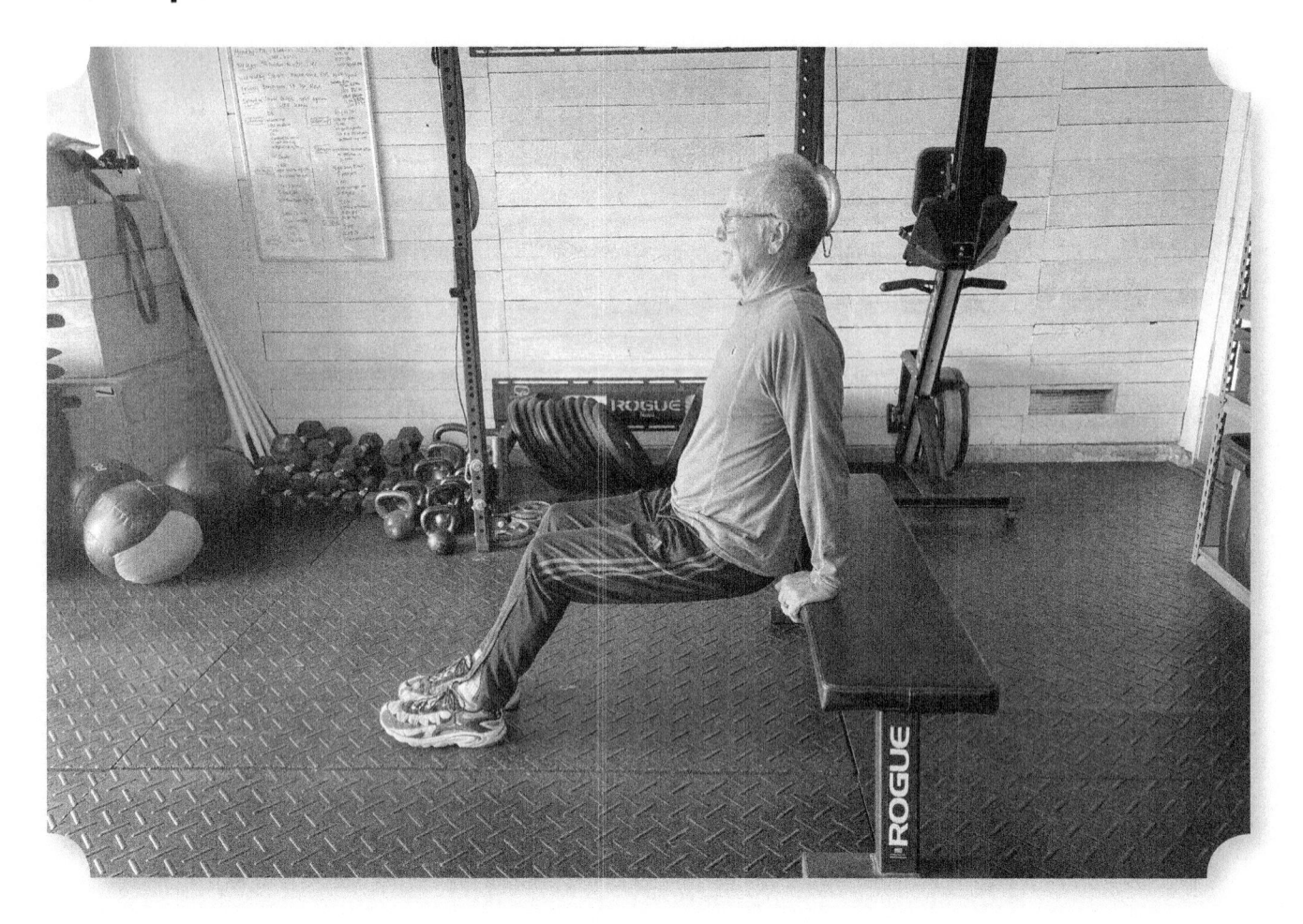

The box dip exercise will strengthen your triceps and upper body. You will need a sturdy box that is about knee height or an exercise bench. Sit on the edge of the bench with your elbows bent and your hands next to your hips, pressing down on the bench. Slide your hips off the box or bench, keeping your feet on the ground. Bend your elbows as you lower your body, stopping when your upper arms are parallel to the ground. Push back up by slowly straightening your arms to the starting position. During the exercise, keep your shoulders down and back, away from your ears, and keep your core muscles engaged to maintain good posture. Start with a small range of motion and gradually increase it as you get stronger. If you have any shoulder or elbow pain, stop the exercise and consult with your healthcare provider before continuing.

Perform 2–3 sets of 10–12 reps, resting for 1–2 minutes between sets. As you get stronger, you can increase the number of sets or reps or try a more challenging variation of the exercise, such as lifting one leg off the ground.

Variations for the Mobility-Impaired

- Chair dip: This is a similar exercise to the box dip, but it uses a chair instead. Sit on the edge of a sturdy chair, place your hands on the edge of the seat on either side of your hips, and slide your body off the chair. Lower yourself down by bending your elbows, then push yourself back up to the starting position.

- Resistance band-assisted dips if you have access to a dip station: Use a resistance band to assist with your dips. Loop the band over the handles of a dip station and put your feet on the other end of the band. This will help take some of the weight off your arms and shoulders, allowing you to perform the exercise with greater ease.

Lateral Raise

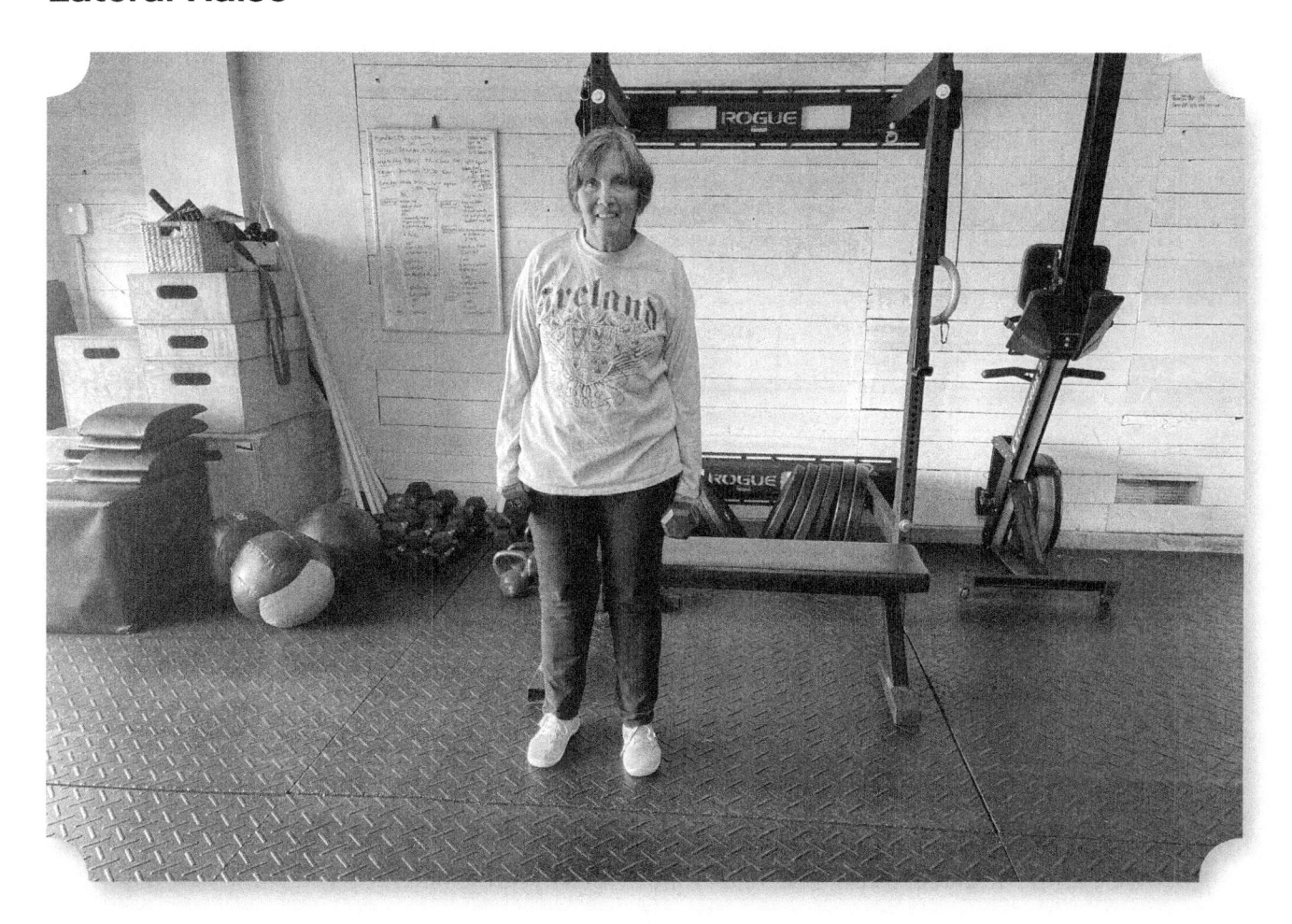

Lateral raises are an ideal exercise to strengthen your shoulders and improve your posture. If you are a beginner, start with light weights, such as 1–2-pound dumbbells, and gradually increase the weight as you get stronger. Start by standing with your feet shoulder-width apart and your knees slightly bent. Hold the weights at your sides with your palms facing your body. Slowly raise your arms out to the sides, keeping your elbows slightly bent, until your arms are parallel to the ground. Hold for a second, then slowly lower your arms back to your sides. It's important to move slowly and avoid jerky movements to help prevent injury and maximize the benefits of the exercise. Start with one set of 10–15 repetitions and gradually increase the number of sets and repetitions as you get stronger.

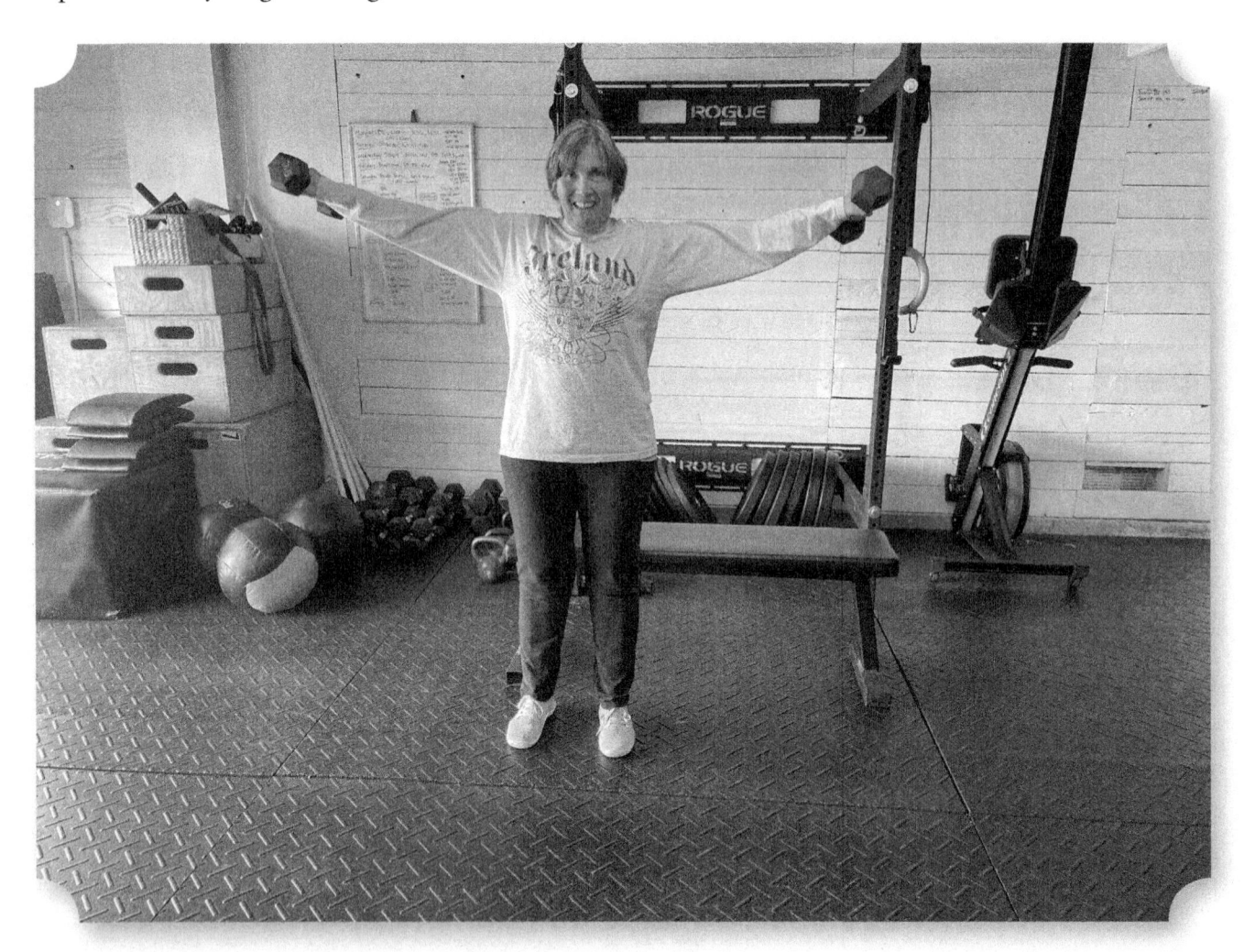

Variations for the Mobility-Impaired

- Seated lateral raise: This variation is similar to the traditional lateral raise, but it can be performed while seated to provide additional stability. Sit on a chair with your feet flat on the ground and a dumbbell in each hand. Raise your arms out to the side, keeping your elbows slightly bent, until they reach shoulder height. Lower the weights back down to the starting position.

- Wall angels: This exercise is a great alternative to lateral raises and is perfect for those with mobility impairments. Stand with your back against a wall with your feet about six inches away from the wall. Bend your elbows to a 90-degree angle with your upper arms against the wall. Slowly raise your arms above your head, keeping your elbows and upper arms against the wall, then lower your arms back down to the starting position.

- Resistance band lateral raise: This variation uses a resistance band instead of dumbbells to perform the exercise. Hold one end of the band in each hand with your arms by your sides. Raise your arms out to the side, keeping your elbows slightly bent, until they reach shoulder height. Lower the band back down to the starting position.

Hip Bridge

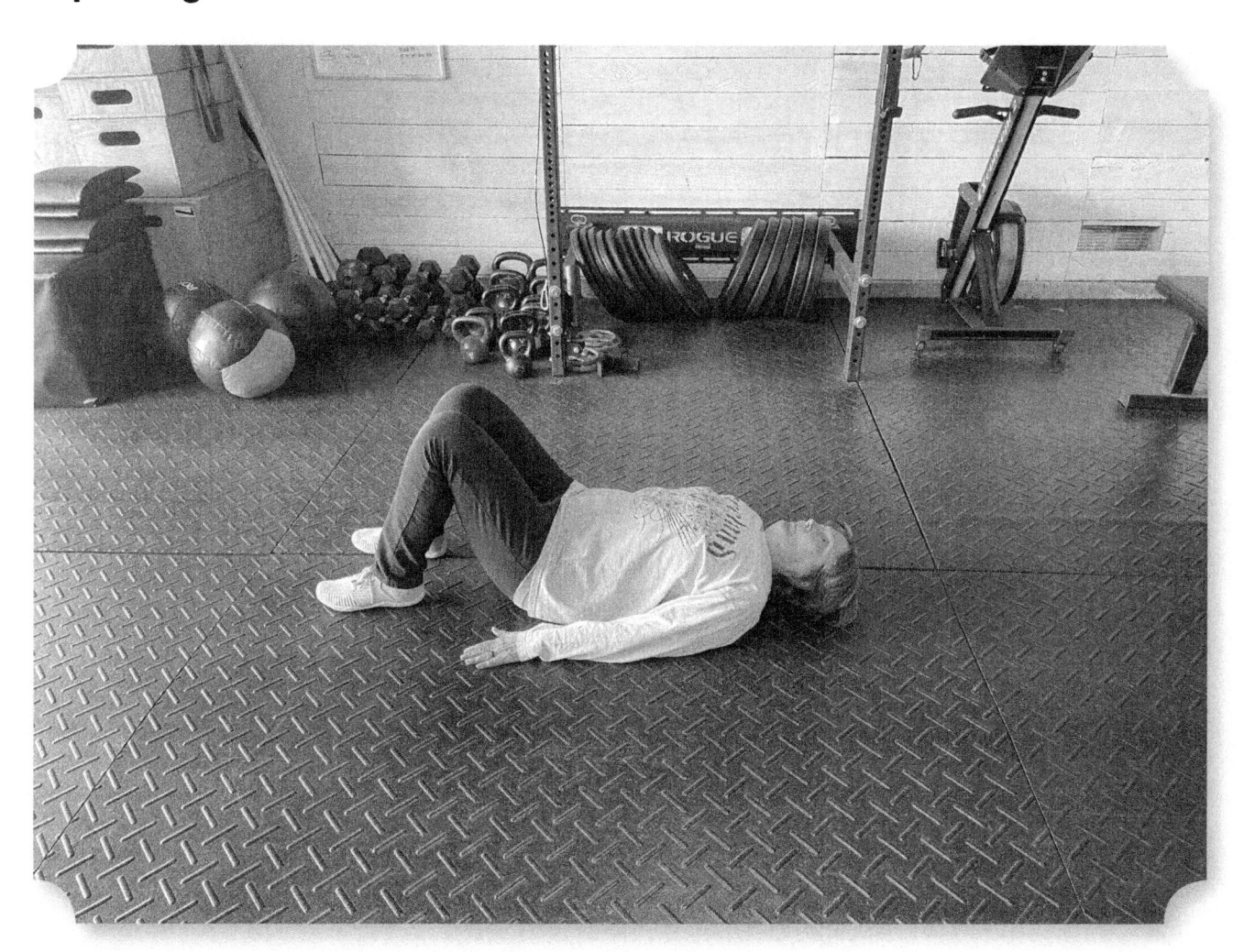

Hip bridges are an efficient exercise to improve strength and mobility in your hips, glutes, and lower back. If you are a beginner, start slowly and gradually increase the intensity and frequency of the exercise over time. Lie on your back on a mat with your knees bent and your feet flat on the floor. Your arms should be by your sides with your palms facing down. Tighten your core muscles by pulling your belly button toward your spine. Slowly lift your hips up toward the ceiling, squeezing your glutes and keeping your knees in line with your hips. Your shoulders, arms, and feet should remain on the ground. Hold the position for a few seconds, then slowly lower your hips back down to the ground. Repeat the exercise 10–15 times or as many as you can comfortably perform.

As you get stronger, you can increase the intensity of the exercise by adding resistance with a resistance band or dumbbells. You can also try single-leg hip bridges to challenge your balance and stability.

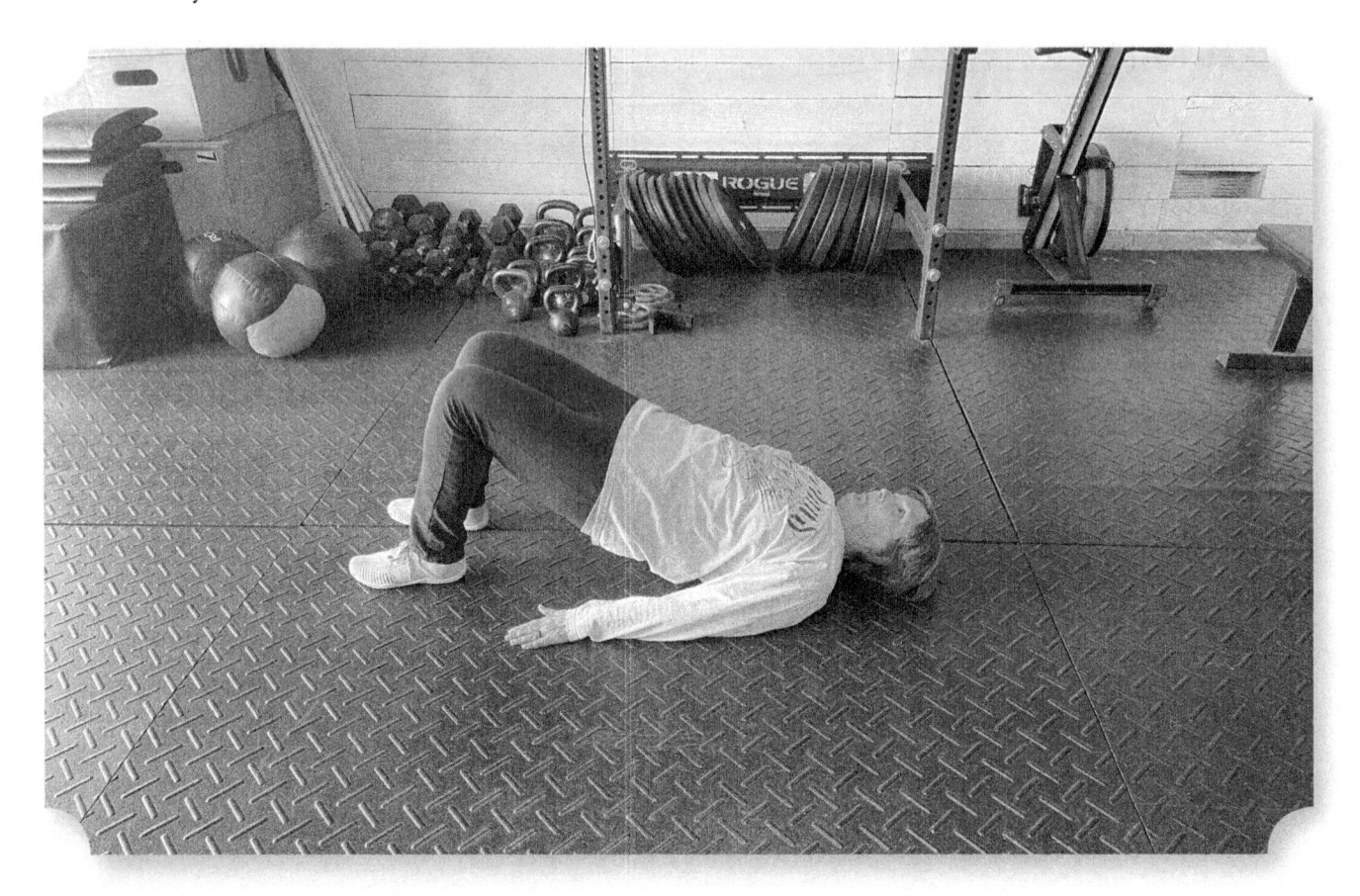

Variations for the Mobility-Impaired

If you have mobility impairments that make it difficult to perform traditional hip bridges, there are a few modifications and variations you can try:

- Wall hip bridge: This variation is a great alternative to traditional hip bridges and can be performed against a wall for added stability. Lie on your back with your feet flat against the wall and your knees bent at a 90-degree angle. Raise your hips off the ground, squeezing your glutes, and hold for a few seconds before lowering your hips back down to the starting position.

- Single-leg hip bridge: This variation is similar to the traditional hip bridge, but it's performed with one leg raised off the ground. Lie on your back with your knees bent and your feet flat on the ground. Lift one foot off the ground, keeping your knee bent, and lift your hips off the ground, squeezing your glutes. Hold for a few seconds before lowering your hips back down to the starting position, then switch legs.

- Seated hip abduction: This exercise focuses on the muscles on your outer thighs and can be done while seated for added stability. Sit on a chair with your feet flat on the ground and a resistance band looped around your ankles. Slowly move your legs apart, stretching the resistance band, then slowly bring your legs back together.

Kettlebell Swing

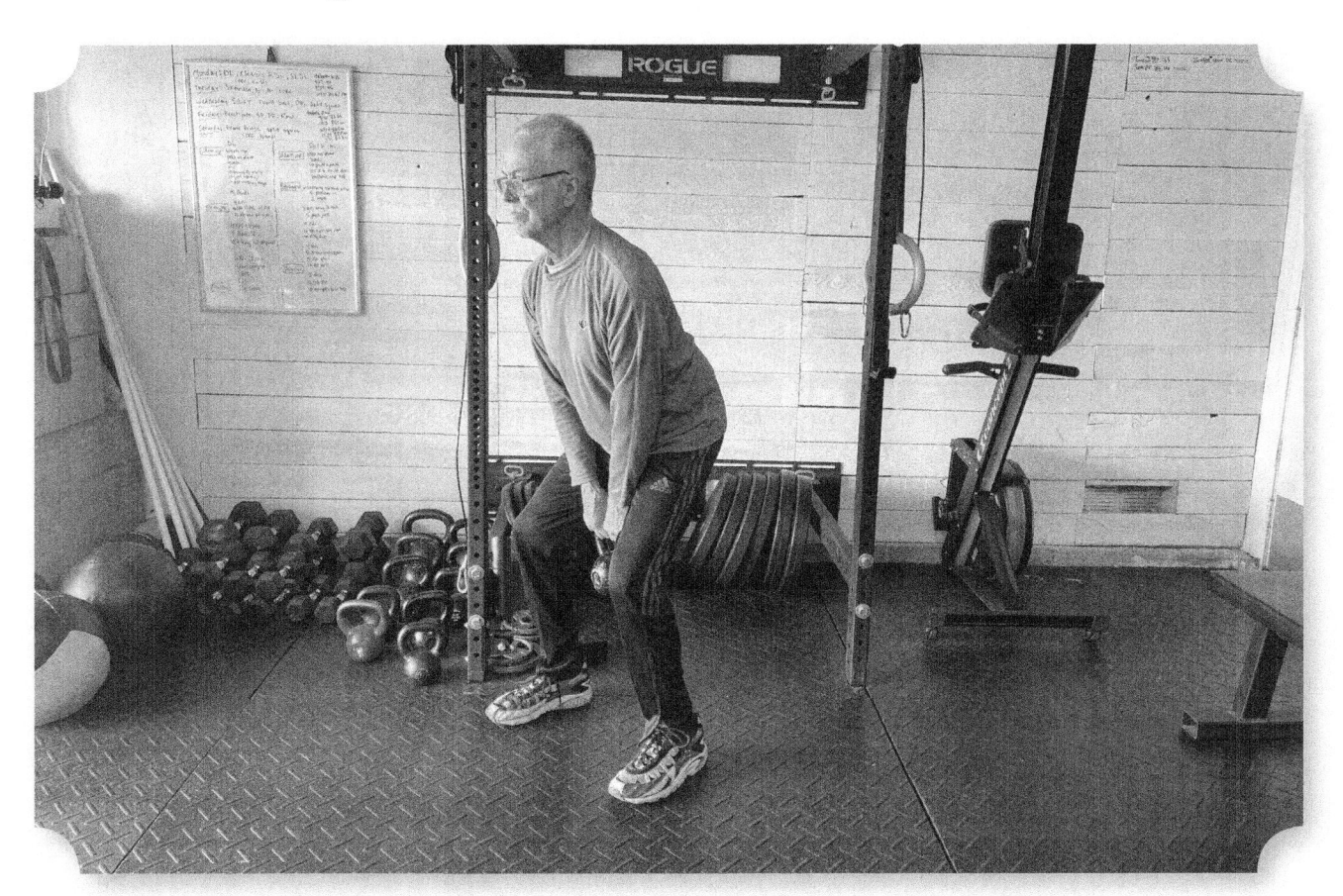

Kettlebell swings will improve strength, balance, and cardiovascular fitness. However, it is important to start with a light weight and gradually increase the load as you become comfortable with the movement. To safely and effectively perform kettlebell swings, start with a kettlebell weight of around 5–10 pounds. Proper form is crucial when performing kettlebell swings to avoid injury. Keep your back straight, hinge at the hips, and use your legs to generate the power to swing the kettlebell. Avoid rounding your back or bending your knees too much. When performing kettlebell swings, make sure you use a full range of motion, bringing the kettlebell all the way up to shoulder level and back down between your legs. Inhale as you swing the kettlebell back between your legs and exhale as you swing it up to shoulder level. If you are a beginner, start with five repetitions and gradually increase the number of repetitions as you become more comfortable with the movement.

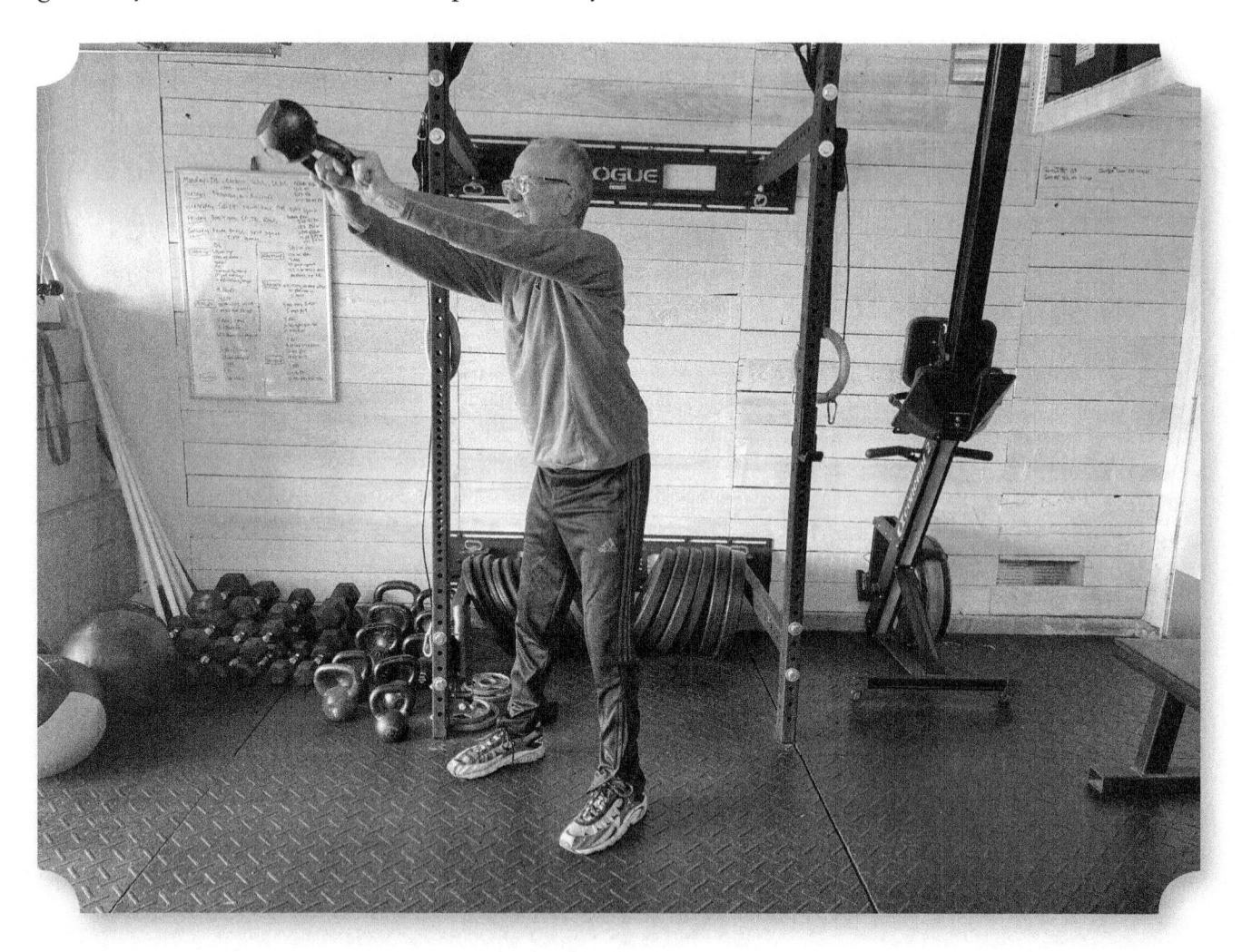

Variations for the Mobility-Impaired

If you have mobility impairments that make it difficult to perform traditional kettlebell swings, there are a few modifications and variations you can try:

- Seated kettlebell swing: This variation is a great alternative to traditional kettlebell swings and can be performed while seated for added stability. Sit on a bench or chair with your feet flat on the ground and a kettlebell in between your legs. Using both hands, pick up the kettlebell and swing it between your legs then up to shoulder height. Repeat for the desired number of repetitions.

- One-arm kettlebell swing: This variation is similar to the traditional kettlebell swing, but it's performed with one arm at a time. Hold the kettlebell in one hand and swing it between your legs then up to shoulder height. Repeat for the desired number of reps, then switch to the other arm.

- Resistance band kettlebell swing: This variation uses a resistance band instead of a kettlebell to perform the exercise. Loop the resistance band under your feet and hold the ends of the band with your hands. Swing your hands back between your legs then forward to shoulder height, squeezing your glutes at the top of the movement.

Plank

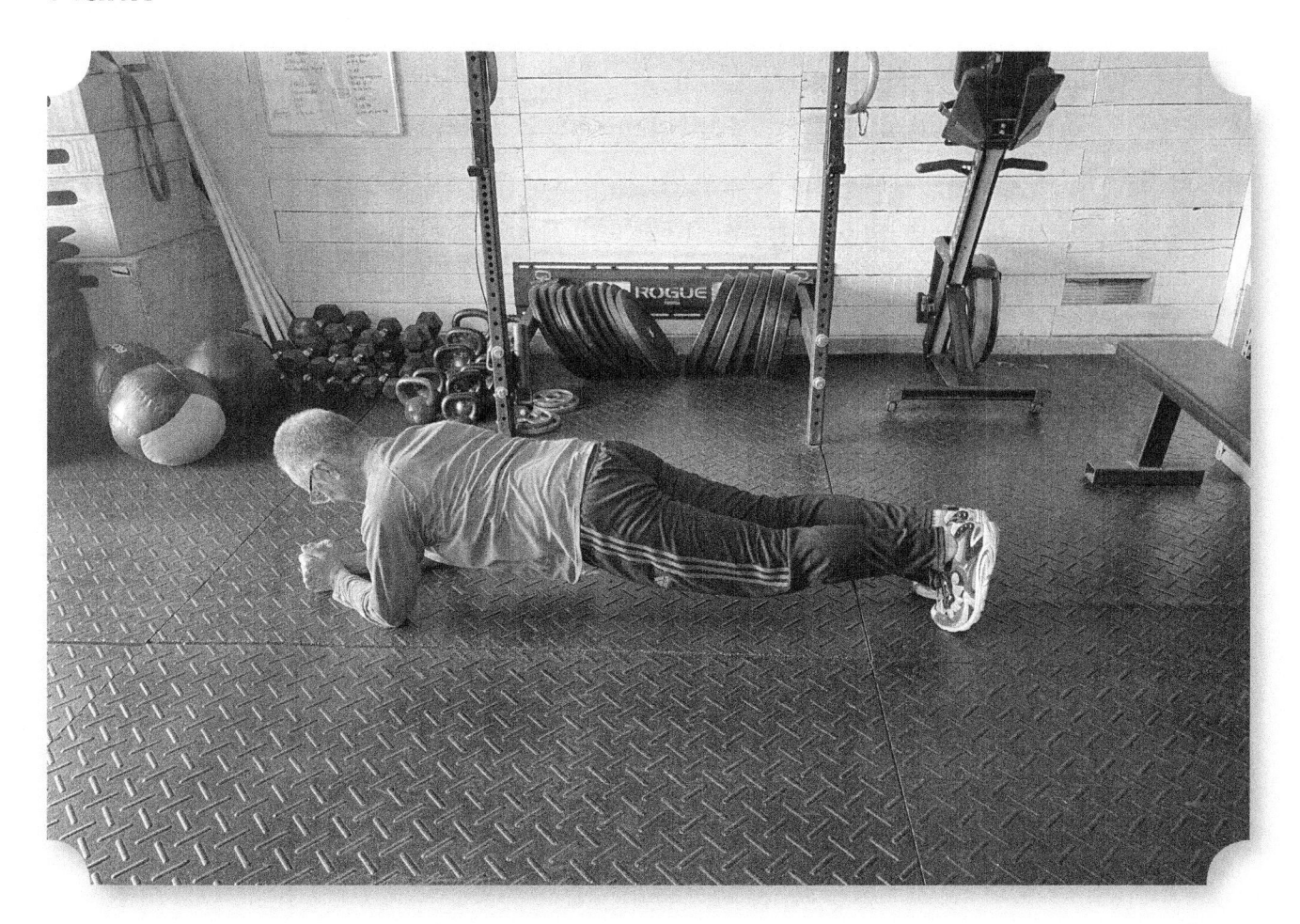

Planks build core strength and stability. Begin by kneeling on the floor and placing your hands on the ground in front of you shoulder-width apart. Slowly step one foot back, followed by the other, until you are in a full plank position. Your hands should be directly under your shoulders, and your body should form a straight line from your head to your heels. Pull your belly button in toward your spine to engage your core muscles. This will help keep your body stable and prevent your lower back from sagging. Hold the plank for a few seconds: Start by holding the plank for 10–15 seconds and gradually work up to longer durations as you get stronger. Be sure to breathe deeply and evenly throughout the exercise. When you're ready to come out of the plank, slowly lower your knees to the ground and rest for a few moments before repeating.

Variations for the Mobility-Impaired

- Wall plank: This variation is a great alternative to traditional planks and can be performed against a wall for added stability. Stand facing a wall with your hands resting on it at shoulder height. Step back with your feet until your body is in a straight line, then hold for the desired amount of time.

- Forearm plank on knees: This variation is similar to the traditional plank, but it's performed on your knees for added stability. Start on your hands and knees, then lower down onto your forearms with your elbows directly under your shoulders. Extend your legs behind you and hold your body in a straight line, engaging your core muscles.

- Side plank on knee: This variation is a modified version of the traditional side plank, and it's performed on your knees for added stability. Start by lying on your side with your bottom knee bent and resting on the ground and your top leg straight. Prop yourself up on your bottom forearm, then lift your hips off the ground, creating a straight line from your shoulders to your knees.

- Plank on an elevated surface: This variation is similar to the traditional plank, but it's performed with your hands on an elevated surface, such as a bench or step. Place your hands on the elevated surface and extend your legs behind you, holding your body in a straight line.

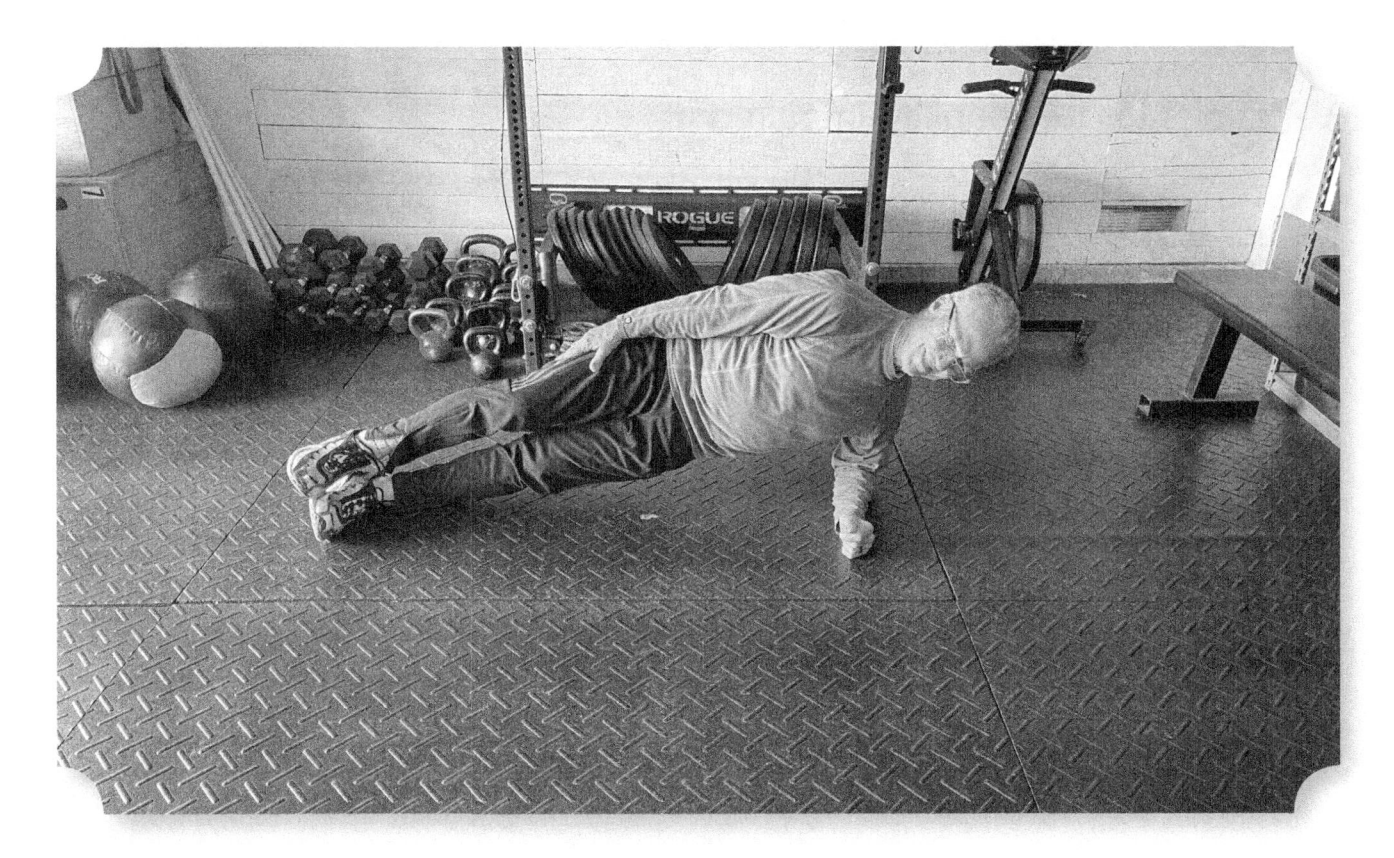

Side Plank

Side planks will strengthen your core, improve balance and stability, and reduce the risk of falls. Start by lying on your side with your legs straight and your feet together. Prop your body up on your elbow, making sure your elbow is directly under your shoulder. Engage your core muscles and lift your hips off the ground, creating a straight line from your head to your heels. Hold the position for 10–30 seconds or as long as you can maintain good form. Bring your hips back down to the ground and repeat on the other side. If you have any shoulder or elbow pain, you can modify the exercise by propping your body up on your hand instead of your elbow. If the full side plank is too difficult, you can start with a modified side plank by bending your bottom knee and propping yourself up on your knee and forearm. As you become stronger, you can increase the hold time and the number of repetitions.

You can add variations to your side plank as your strength increases, such as:

- Side plank with leg lift: This variation adds a leg lift to the traditional side plank. Start in a traditional side plank position with your body in a straight line. Lift your top leg up and hold for a few seconds, then lower it back down. Switch sides and repeat.

- Side plank with arm reach: This variation adds an arm reach to the traditional side plank. Start in a traditional side plank position with your body in a straight line. Reach your top arm up toward the ceiling, then bring it back down. Hold the position for five seconds, then switch sides. Gradually increase the amount of time holding the position.

Variations for the Mobility-Impaired

If you have mobility impairments that make it difficult to perform traditional side planks, there are a few modifications and variations you can try:

- Side plank on knee: This variation is a modified version of the traditional side plank, and it's performed on your knee for added stability. Start by lying on your side with your bottom knee bent and resting on the ground and your top leg straight. Prop yourself up on your bottom forearm, then lift your hips off the ground, creating a straight line from your shoulders to your knees.

- Side plank on an elevated surface: This variation is similar to the traditional side plank, but it's performed with your hand on an elevated surface, such as a bench or step. Place your hand on the elevated surface and extend your legs behind you, holding your body in a straight line.

Leg Lifts

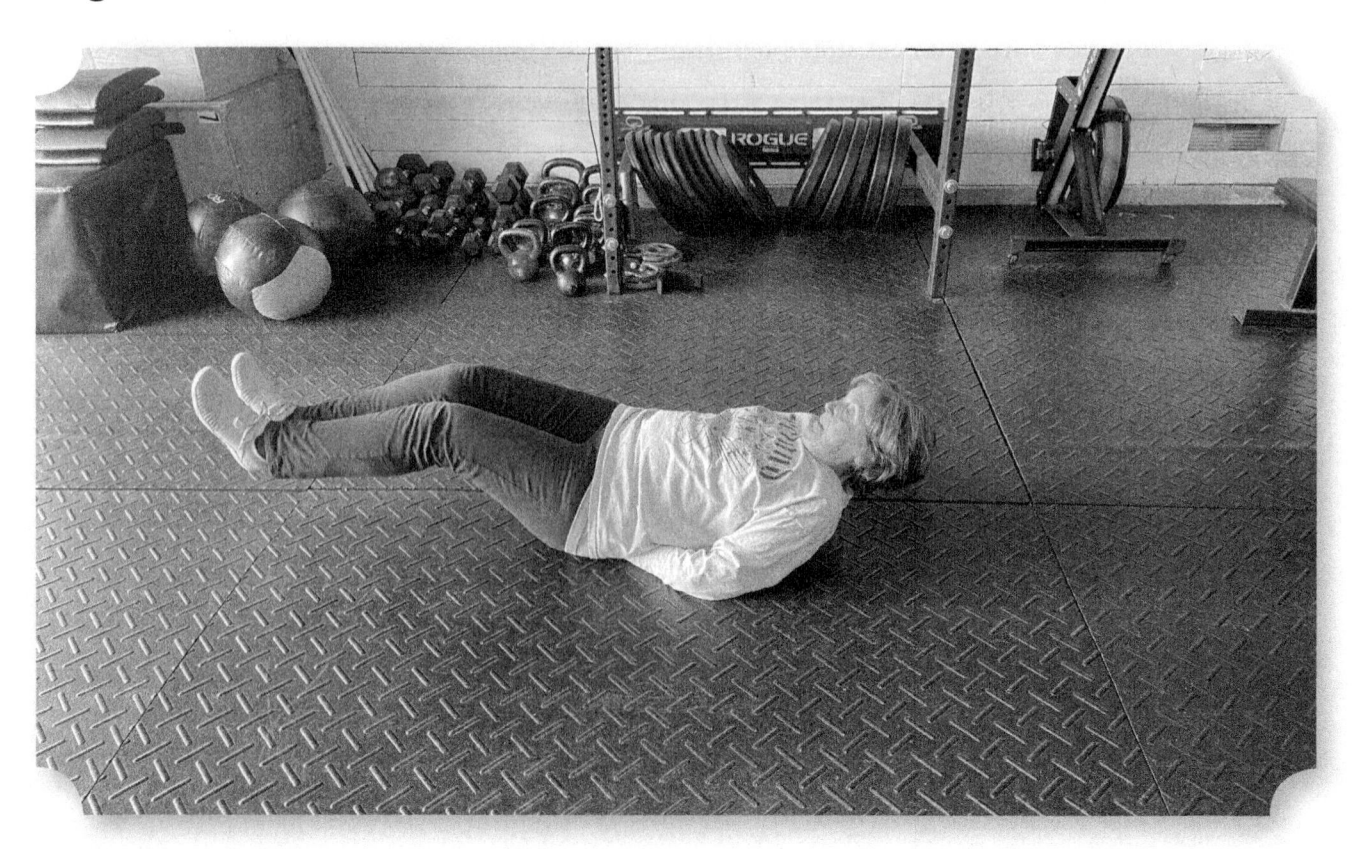

Leg lifts strengthen your core and lower body muscles. Start this exercise by lying down on your back with your legs straight and your arms tucked under your glutes. Slowly lift your legs off the ground, bending your knees slightly. Hold your legs up for a few seconds, then slowly lower them back down. Do 5–10 repetitions if you are a beginner. Gradually add repetitions and sets. If you are new to strength training, start with low lifts and gradually increase the range of motion as your strength improves.

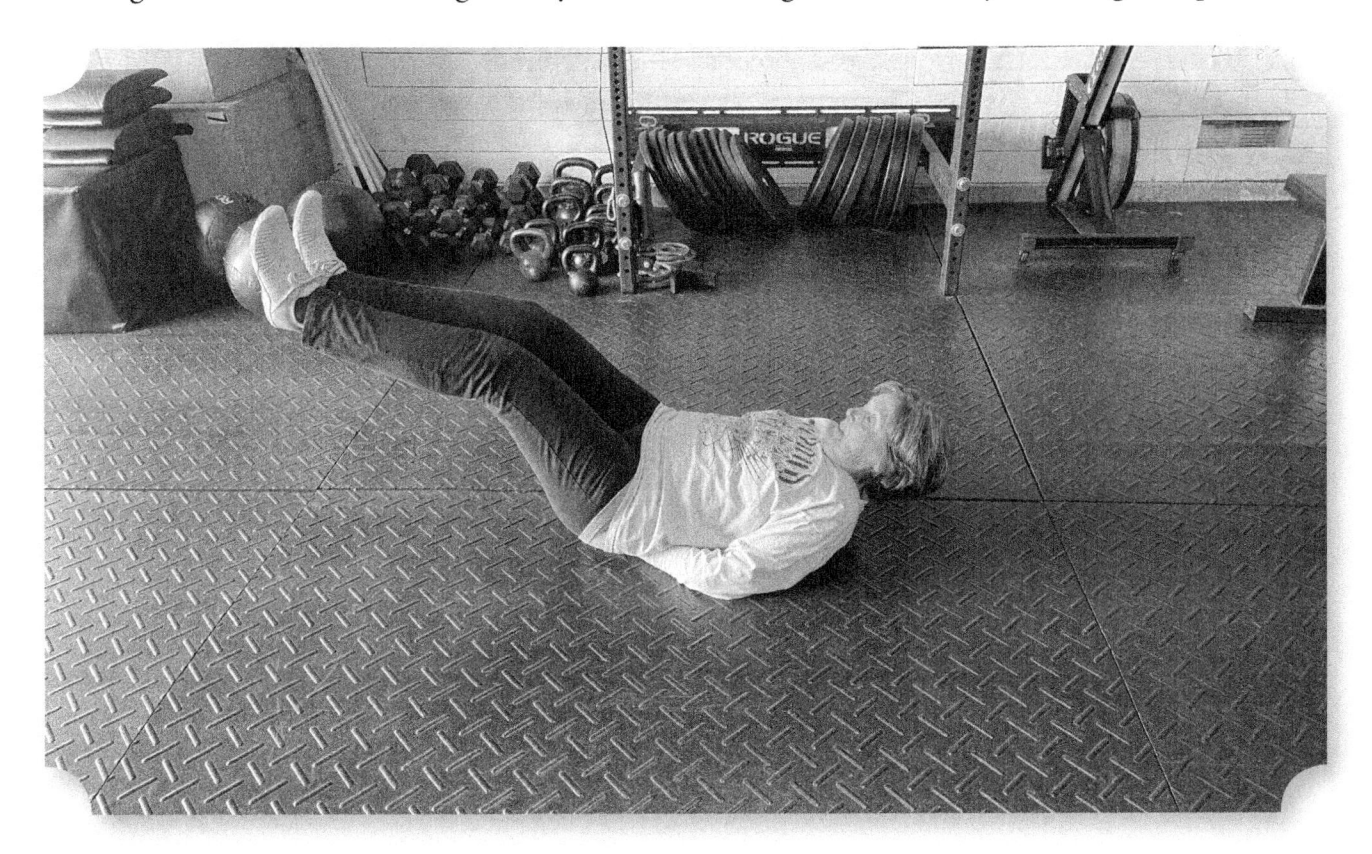

Variations for the Mobility-Impaired

If you have mobility impairments that make it difficult to perform traditional leg lifts, there are a few modifications and variations you can try:

- Seated leg lifts: This variation is performed while seated on a chair or bench. Sit with your back straight and your feet flat on the ground. Lift one leg up as high as you can, then lower it back down. Repeat five times, then switch legs.

- Lying single-leg lifts with bent knees: This variation is performed lying down with your knees bent. Lie on your back with your knees bent and your feet flat on the ground. Lift one leg up as high as you can, then lower it back down. Repeat for the desired number of reps, then switch legs.

- Wall leg lifts: This variation is performed while standing with your back against a wall for added stability. Stand with your back against a wall and your feet a few inches away from it. Lift one leg up as high as you can, then lower it back down. Repeat for the desired number of reps, then switch legs.

- Seated leg extensions: This variation is performed while seated on a chair or bench. Sit with your back straight and your feet flat on the ground. Lift one leg up and extend it out straight in front of you, then lower it back down. Repeat for the desired number of reps, then switch legs.

Chapter 7:
At-Home Workouts

To start a strength training workout program with high repetitions and heavy weights is to invite injury. Unrealistic expectations can cause you to abandon your goals. The smart way to build strength is to start basic and light and add more repetitions and weight when the exercise isn't challenging anymore. Muscle grows and strengthens according to the principle of progressive overload. This principle means that you will get the best strength gains if you don't increase the time, weight, or intensity of your workout by more than 10% per week (Waehner, n.d.). More overload will lead to injury, and no progressive overload will result in a plateau where you will exercise but not gain more strength.

The following 12 at-home basic workouts are fully scalable to make them accessible for beginners and more challenging for an advanced program. There are four lower-body workouts, four upper-body workouts, and four full-body workouts. If you do two workouts per week, this will give you a six-week program. If you do three workouts per week, you will have a three-week program.

Be aware that these workouts can be repeated once you've gone through them. It will benefit your muscle strength and movement patterns greatly if you repeat the workouts multiple times after going through all 12. This program offers a potential 6–12 weeks of workouts, and you will see a progressive increase in your strength.

Are Home Workouts Better Than a Gym?

The at-home workouts in this book are tailored to take advantage of the benefits of exercising in your own space. Here are some of those benefits:

- Convenience: One of the biggest advantages of working out at home is the convenience it offers. You can exercise whenever you want without having to leave your home or worry about transportation to a gym or fitness class.

- Safety: For seniors who have mobility or balance issues, working out at home can be safer than going to a gym or fitness class. You can exercise at your own pace and in a familiar and comfortable environment, reducing the risk of falls or other injuries.

- Cost savings: Working out at home can be more cost-effective than a gym membership or fitness class. You can start with simple, inexpensive equipment like resistance bands or light weights and gradually add more equipment as you progress.

- Flexibility: Working out at home allows you to be flexible with your exercise routines. You can choose the type of exercise that is best for your individual needs.

- Reduced stress: Working out at home can be less stressful than going to a gym or fitness class. You can exercise in a relaxed, comfortable environment without worrying about social pressures or distractions.

- Improved mental health: Exercise has a positive effect on mental health as it can reduce stress, anxiety, and depression. If you are dealing with isolation or other mental health issues, working out at home can be a helpful way to improve your mood and overall well-being.

At Home Workouts:

The 12 workouts in this book are broken up into 4 lower body workouts, 4 upper body workouts, and 4 full body workouts. Each workout starts with a warm-up which should take between 5-10 minutes. The second part of the workout is the Strength section. This is the body part we are focusing on that day. The movements in the Strength section are pictured and described in the previous chapters above. How you move through the strength section is described in each individual workout. The finisher is the cool-down to the workout.

Lower Body Workout 1

Warm-up:

Do **three rounds** of each of the following exercises to loosen your joints, warm your muscles, and make more oxygen available to your muscles. The warm-up is part of the workout and is not an optional extra if you want the full benefits of strength training.

1. **Walk** outside for a distance of about 200 meters (or for about 2 minutes). If you have a stationary bike, treadmill, or rower, you can use those machines instead of the outdoor walk during the warm-up and cool-down. If walking outside isn't an option, and you don't have access to the machines mentioned above, you can replace the walk with 30 seconds of marching in place to get your heart rate up and your muscles warm.

   You can substitute the 2-minute walk with the 30-second marching for all the warm-ups and cool-downs in the workouts below!

2. **Overhead side-to-side stretch**, 5 times to each side

3. **10 squat-to-chair** exercises

Strength:

Do **five rounds** of the following exercises every 3 minutes and then rest for 3 minutes. If you finish a round before 3 minutes is up, rest the remaining time. If it takes you longer than 3 minutes, you may rest until you feel ready to go to the next round.

1. **10 squat-to-chairs** while holding a dumbbell in each hand at the shoulders

2. **10 step-ups** with each leg to a low box or stair

Do **four rounds** of the following exercises every 3 minutes. Rest for the remaining time if you finish a round before the 3 minutes is over.

1. **10 reverse lunges** with each leg. Stand to the side of a sturdy chair and use it to guide you up and down. Make sure your back knee goes to the ground.

2. **30-second plank**. If you find the standard plank too difficult, you can put your knees on the ground.

Finisher:

Do **three rounds** of the following exercises:

1. **Walk** outside for 2 minutes

2. **5 cat/cow** stretches

3. **30-second hamstring stretch**

Lower Body Workout 2

Warm-Up:

Do **three rounds** of each of the following exercises to increase the blood flow to your muscles:

1. **Walk** outside for 200 m or about 2 minutes

2. **Overhead side-to-side stretches**, 5 stretches to each side

3. **10 pvc deadlifts**

4. **30-second plank** with the knees on the ground

Strength:

Do **five rounds** of the following exercises every 3 minutes. If the work takes less than 3 minutes, use the remaining time to rest before the next round starts.

1. **10 deadlifts** Use a light barbell or a set of dumbbells

2. **10 step-ups** with each leg to a low box or stair

Do **four rounds** of the following exercises every 3 minutes; rest for the remainder of the time if you finish a round before the 3 minutes are over.

1. **10 single-leg deadlifts with each leg**. Hold onto the back of a chair and focus on the balance of the planted leg. Bend forward while maintaining square hips. Don't bend further forward than you can comfortably manage. Use the chair as your guide.

2. **15 leg lifts**, done while lying on the floor

Finisher:

Three rounds of the following exercises to finish:

1. **Walk** outside for 2 minutes

2. **5 cat/cow** stretches

3. **30-second child's pose**

Lower Body Workout 3

Warm-Up:

Three rounds to reduce the risk of injury by starting your workout with the following exercises:

1. **Walk** outside for approximately 2 minutes (200 m)

2. **30-second child's pose**

3. **10 squat-to-chairs**

Strength:

Do **five rounds** of the following exercises every 3 minutes. If the work takes less than 3 minutes, use the remaining time to rest before the next round starts.

1. **10 squat-to-chairs** using a set of dumbbells

2. **10 step-ups with each leg** to a low box or stair (step up and down to a stair, alternating legs for a total of 10 step-ups)

Do **four rounds** of the following exercises every 3 minutes. Rest for the remaining time if you finish a round before the 3 minutes is over.

1. **10–12 hip bridges.** Lie on your back, keeping your knees bent and feet flat on the ground. Lift your hips upward to form a straight line between your shoulders and knees. Squeeze your glutes at the top of the movement and keep your core tight as you raise and lower your hips.

Finisher:

Three rounds to cool your muscles with the following exercises:

1. **Walk** outside for 2 minutes
2. **5 cat/cow stretches**
3. **30-second child's pose**

Lower Body Workout 4

Do **three rounds** of the following to prepare your muscles and joints for strength training:

1. **Walk** outside for approximately 2 minutes (200 m)
2. **30-second child's pose**
3. **10 kettlebell swings**

Strength:

Do **four rounds** of the following exercises every 3 minutes. Rest for the remaining time if you finish the work before the 3 minutes is over.

1. **10 kettlebell deadlifts** with your legs straight
2. **45-second plank** on all fours (with your knees and elbows on the floor)

Do **five rounds** of the following exercises every 3 minutes. If the work takes less than 3 minutes, use the remaining time to rest before the next round starts.

1. **10 deadlifts** using a light barbell or a set of dumbbells
2. **10 step-ups to a low box or stair** (step up and down to a stair, alternating legs for a total of 10 step-ups)

Core:

1. Do **three rounds of 15 leg lifts**; rest as needed between the sets.

Finisher:

Three rounds. Bring your body back to a resting state by doing the following exercises:

1. **Walk** outside for 2 minutes
2. 5 cat/cow stretches
3. 30-second child's pose

Upper Body Workout 1

Warm-Up:

Three rounds: Increase the blood flow to your muscles by doing the following exercises:

1. **Walk** outside for 200 m or approximately 2 minutes
2. **Overhead side-to-side stretch**, 5 stretches to each side
3. **10 squat-to-chairs**
4. **30-second plank** with your knees and elbows on the floor

Strength:

Five rounds: Train your muscles by doing every 2 minutes:

1. **10 overhead presses** with dumbbells, then rest for another round of 2 minutes.

Four rounds every 2.5 minutes of the following:

1. **10 dumbbell bicep curls**
2. **10 dumbbell lateral raises**

Do **three rounds** every 2.5 minutes of the following:

1. **10 box dips**
2. **10 dumbbell hammer curls** (hold the dumbbells vertically)

Finisher:

Do **three rounds** of the following exercises to return your heart rate to the resting state:

1. **Walk** outside for 2 minutes
2. **10 leg lifts**
3. **5 cat/cow** stretches

Upper Body Workout 2

Warm-up:

Three rounds: Increase the available oxygen to your muscles by doing the following exercises:

1. **Walk outside** for 200 m (approximately 2 minutes)
2. **Overhead side-to-side stretch**, 5 times to each side
3. **10 squat-to-chairs**
4. **10 knee push-ups** (scale to hands on wall or hands on a 24-in. height chair/box)

Strength:

Five rounds: Build your strength and stamina by completing every 3 minutes of the following exercises, then rest the remaining 3 minutes:

1. **10 kettlebell swings**
2. **10 chest presses** on the floor with dumbbells

Do **four rounds** every 2.5 minutes of the following exercises:

1. **10 single-arm rows on a box or chair**, 10 rows with each arm
2. **30-second plank** with your knees on the floor

Do **three rounds** every 1.5 minutes:

1. **10 push-ups on your knees** with hands on a chair, the wall, or even the ground.

Finisher:

Three rounds: Return your body to the resting state by doing the following exercises:

1. **Walk** outside for 2 minutes
2. **10 squat-to-chairs**
3. **5 cat/cow** stretches
4. **30-second child's pose**

Upper Body Workout 3

Warm-Up:

Three rounds: Prepare your body for your workout by completing the following exercises:

1. **Walk** outside for 2 minutes (200 m)
2. **Overhead side-to-side stretch**, 5 times to each side
3. **10 squat-to-chairs**
4. **10 kettlebell swings**

Strength:

Five rounds every 2 minutes:

1. **10 overhead presses** with dumbbells every 2 minutes; rest the time it takes to finish the presses until the next round of 2 minutes starts.

Four rounds every 3 minutes of the following:

1. **10 dumbbell bicep curls**
2. **10 dumbbell lateral raises**
3. **30-second plank** with your knees on the ground

Three rounds every 2.5 minutes

1. **10 box dips**
2. **10 leg lifts on the floor**

Round off your strength training with:

Three rounds every minute of:

1. **15 standing dumbbell bicep curls.**

Finisher:

Do **three rounds** of the following exercises:

1. **Walk** outside for 2 minutes

2. **10 stair step-ups**

3. **5 cat/cow** stretches

Upper Body Workout 4

Warm-Up:

Do **three rounds** of the following exercises to prepare your muscles and joints for strength training:

1. **Walk** outside for 2 minutes or 200 m

2. **Overhead side-to-side stretch**, 5 stretches to each side

3. **10 kettlebell swings**

4. **10 push-ups to box**, knees on the ground

Strength:

Do **five rounds** every 2 minutes of:

1. **10 standing bent-over rows with both feet on the ground.** You can hold a barbell or a dumbbell in each hand.

Do **four rounds** every 2.5 minutes of the following exercises:

1. **10 dumbbell chest presses** from the ground

2. **10 hip bridges** on the ground

3. **10 single-arm rows on each arm** with a dumbbell or a kettlebell with your knee on a chair, box, or bench

Finisher:

Cool down with **three rounds** of these exercises:

1. **Walk** outside for 2 minutes

2. **10 leg lifts**

3. **5 cat/cow** stretches

Full Body Workout 1

Warm-Up:

Get your circulation going with **three rounds** of the following exercises:

1. **Walk** outside for 200 m or about 2 minutes

2. **Overhead side-to-side stretches**, 5 stretches to each side

3. **10 squat-to-chairs**

4. **10 push-ups, knees on the ground**. Scale by putting knees on the ground and pushing against the wall or hands on the top of a chair or bench.

Strength:

Five rounds every 3 minutes: If the work takes less than 3 minutes, use the remaining time to rest before the next round starts.

1. **10 single-leg deadlifts, 10 deadlifts on each leg**. Hold onto the back of a chair or wall and work on the balance of the planted leg. Bend forward and maintain square hips; only bend as far as you can. Use the chair as your guide.

2. **10 kettlebell swings**

Do **four rounds** every 2.5 minutes of these exercises:

1. **10 push-ups to box on knees**

2. **10 single-arm bent-over rows with dumbbells**

End off your strength routine with **three rounds** every 2.5 minutes of these exercises:

1. **10 squat-to-box** exercises, holding a weight at your chest

2. **30-second plank**; you can keep your knees on the ground

Finisher:

Cool your muscles with **three rounds** of the following:

1. **Walking** outside for 2 minutes

2. **10 leg lifts**

3. **5 cat/cow** stretches

Full Body Workout 2

Warm-Up:

Start your workout with **three rounds** of the following exercises:

1. **Walk** outside for 200 m, or approximately 2 minutes

2. **Overhead side-to-side stretch**, 5 stretches to each side

3. **10 squat-to-chairs**

4. **10 leg lifts**

5. **10 push-ups to a box or chair** with your knees on the ground

Strength:

Develop your strength with **five rounds** of these exercises every 3 minutes. If the work takes less than 3 minutes, use the remaining time to rest before the next round starts.

1. **10 squat-to-box or bench**, holding dumbbells on your shoulders

2. **10 kettlebell swings**

Do **four rounds** every 2.5 minutes of the following exercises:

1. **20 reverse lunges, 10 lunges on each leg**. Hold the back of the chair for support and only lower yourself down as low as you can get up from.

2. **10 step-ups onto stairs or a low box**

Do **four rounds** every 2.5 minutes of the following:

1. **10 box dips**

2. **10 sitting dumbbell shoulder presses**

Finisher:

Minimize delayed onset soreness with a cool-down of **3 rounds** of:

1. **Walking** outside for 2 minutes

2. **30-second plank on the ground**; you can use your knees

3. **5 cat/cow** stretches

Full Body Workout 3

Warm-Up:

Loosen up your muscles and joints with **3 rounds** of these exercises:

1. **Walk** outside for 200 m, or approximately 2 minutes

2. **Overhead side-to-side stretch**, 5 stretches to each side

3. **10 squat-to-chairs**

4. **10 shoulder presses with light weights**

5. **10 kettlebell swings**

Strength:

Challenge your muscles with **five rounds** of the following exercises every 3 minutes. If the work takes less than 3 minutes, use the remaining time to rest before the next round starts.

1. **10 straight-leg deadlifts** with kettlebells or a set of dumbells
2. **10 hip bridges**

Do **four rounds** every 2.5 minutes of these exercises:

1. **10 standing dumbbell lateral raises**
2. **10 step-ups using stairs or a low box**

Complete **four rounds** every 2.5 minutes of the following:

1. **10 sitting bicep curls**
2. **10 sitting dumbbell shoulder presses**, one arm at a time

Finisher:

Relax your muscles by doing **three rounds** of these finishers:

1. **Walk** outside for 2 minutes
2. **10 leg lifts**
3. **5 cat/cow** stretches

Full Body Workout 4

Warm-Up:

Increase the blood flow to your muscles with **three rounds** of these exercises:

1. **Walk** outside for 200 m, or approximately 2 minutes
2. **Overhead side-to-side stretch**, 5 times to each side
3. **10 squat-to-chairs**
4. **10 leg lifts**
5. **10 standing dumbbell lateral raises**

Strength:

Increase your strength with **five rounds** of the following exercises every 3 minutes. If the work takes less than 3 minutes, use the remaining time to rest before the next round starts.

1. **10 thrusters** (squat-to-chair or box, then shoulder press when you move up to a standing position)
2. **30-second plank on the ground**; you can put your knees on the floor

Complete **four rounds** every 2.5 minutes of these exercises:

1. **20 reverse lunges, 10 lunges on each leg**. Use the back of a sturdy, nonslip chair for support, and only lower yourself as low as you can get up from.
2. **10 kettlebell swings**

Strengthen your arms by doing **four rounds** every 2.5 minutes of the following:

1. **10 standing bicep curls**
2. **10 box dips**

Finisher:

Ease out of your workout by doing **three rounds** of the following:

1. **Walk** outside for 2 minutes
2. **10 squat-to-chairs**
3. **5 cat/cow** stretches

I hope you like these workouts and find them doable, but challenging! Remember you can scale any workout to make them easier. Do less rounds or fewer reps and build up to the work that is in the workouts. On the other hand, you can make the workouts more challenging by raising your weight or adding more reps! You can also make the body weight movements more challenging as you get stronger!

Using the Daily Workout and Healthy Habits Log

An exercise log is a great tool to help you track your physical activity and fitness progress over time. Adding your notes about hydration, dietary protein, and sleep will help you keep an eye on your progress toward your new healthy habits. Before you start tracking your exercise, set some goals for yourself. What do you want to achieve with your fitness routine? Do you have a specific weakness you want to remedy, such as weak leg muscles? Do you want to be able to carry your own groceries?

When you have decided on your goals, use the Daily Workout and Healthy Habits Log provided in this chapter to:

- Record your exercise. Every time you exercise, record the details in your exercise log. This should include the type of exercise, the number of sets and repetitions, and your heart rate directly after doing the exercise.

- Track your progress. Regularly review your exercise log to see how you are progressing toward your goals. Look for patterns in your exercise routine and see if there are areas where you need to make changes or adjustments.

- Adjust your routine. Use the information in your exercise log to make adjustments to your exercise routine. If you are not seeing the results you want, try changing the type or intensity of your exercise. If you are consistently meeting or exceeding your goals, challenge yourself to set new ones.

- Stay consistent. Consistency is key when it comes to exercise. Use your exercise log to help you stay on track and make exercise a regular part of your daily routine.

By using an exercise log, you can stay motivated and focused on your fitness goals, track your progress, and make adjustments to your exercise routine as needed.

If you are able, make a photocopy of the Daily Workout and Healthy Habits Log provided on the next page, so you can track your workouts and healthy habits for multiple days!

Daily Workout & Healthy Habits Log

WARM UP

Exercise	Set	Rep	Heart Rate

STRENGTH TRAINING

Exercise	Set	Rep	Heart Rate

STRENGTH TRAINING

Exercise	Set	Rep	Heart Rate

DAILY HABITS

EXERCISE	WATER	PROTEIN	SLEEP

Chapter 8:
Nutrition and Healthy Habits

Healthy habits are part of a lifestyle. They form an essential part of a long-term strategy for optimal health, longevity, independence, and quality of life. They are gifts to your future self.

Nutrition

Nutrition is just as important as exercise—maybe even more so. As we age, our dietary needs change, and we have to be aware of these changes to adapt our meals accordingly. Do away with junk food and have nutrient-dense foods on the table instead. A nutrient-dense food has a high vitamin and mineral content and usually was pulled from the ground or plucked from a tree. Such food often has a bright color, which is nature's way of signifying a healthy, nutritious meal.

As you start exercising, you'll find that you might be hungrier during the day. This is normal and a good sign that your body is building more muscle and speeding up your metabolism. It is important to fuel your body with good carbohydrates such as potatoes, oatmeal, whole-grain bread and pasta, and fresh fruits and vegetables (eat the rainbow). Fuel your muscles with protein from chicken, fish, turkey, steak, Greek yogurt, cheese, and milk. Feed your cell membranes with healthy fats contained in nuts, avocados, and olive oil.

Monitoring your blood sugar level is important for optimal energy levels. Eating prior to a workout will make energy available to your muscles. Nourish yourself after a workout to maintain your energy. Avoid foods that have a high sugar content to maintain a stable blood sugar level.

A Little More About Nutrients

Macronutrients (carbs, fats, and protein) are needed by your body in large amounts. During digestion, most carbs are broken down into sugar molecules called glucose. Your brain, red blood cells, and central nervous system use glucose for fuel. Muscles and the liver store glucose to release when your body demands energy. If you follow a low-carb diet, your body will also use fats and protein for energy. Fiber is a type of carb that can't be digested by humans. Our digestive system needs fiber to keep our bowel movements regular and to feel full after eating.

Protein becomes of paramount importance as we age since it prevents the loss of muscle mass. Protein fuels our muscles and forms the building blocks of muscles, skin, bones, and organs. Our bodies use protein for cell repair and maintenance and to make enzymes and hormones. Our immune systems depend on proteins to make antibodies and help heal wounds.

Fats are used by your body as an energy reserve. If you burn fewer calories than you take in, the extra calories will be stored as fat. While excess fat is unhealthy, your body needs fat to protect your organs, facilitate the absorption of fat-soluble vitamins, and build cell membranes.

Micronutrients are vitamins and minerals. There are 13 vitamins and 13 minerals that your body can't make by itself and has to get from your diet. They are called essential vitamins and minerals. Your body can produce a certain amount of vitamins D, K, B12, and B7 (biotin). Vitamins are sourced from plants and animals, and minerals from soil and water.

There are two types of vitamins: fat-soluble and water-soluble. Vitamins that can be dissolved in water (water-soluble) include

- vitamin B1 (thiamine), which helps the body convert nutrients into energy.

- vitamin B2 (riboflavin), is essential for proper cell function, the metabolism of fats, and to help produce energy.

- vitamin B3 (niacin), necessary to change food into energy.

- vitamin B5 (pantothenic acid), is needed for the synthesis of fatty acids.

- vitamin B6 (pyridoxine), which plays a role during the release of glucose from stored carbohydrates and during the creation of red blood cells.

- vitamin B7 (biotin), is used during the metabolism of glucose, fatty acids, and amino acids.

- vitamin B9 (folate), essential for cell division.

- vitamin B12 (cobalamin), which is needed for creating red blood cells and for proper brain function.

- vitamin C (ascorbic acid) is used to create collagen (the protein that keeps the skin elastic and forms a component of tendons, ligaments, and the cornea) and assists with the healing of wounds. It is also vital for healthy bones and blood vessels, plays a part in the absorption of iron, and is an antioxidant.

Fat-soluble vitamins include

- vitamin A, which is needed for maintaining the light-sensitive cells in the eyes and the proper functioning of mucous membranes, and it plays an important role in hair and cell growth.

- vitamin D, is required for the absorption of calcium and phosphorus during digestion, a strong immune system, and proper mineralization of the bones. Your body needs sunlight to make vitamin D.

- vitamin E, which is an antioxidant that protects your body against damage by free radicals.

- vitamin K, used by the liver to make blood clotting agents. It also helps to prevent blood vessels from being calcified and is essential for healthy bones.

Timing of Meals and Snacks for Optimal Performance

The timing of your meals and snacks is important for optimal performance and recovery. Here are some guidelines:

- Eat a pre-workout meal or snack 1–2 hours before your workout. This should be a balanced meal with protein, carbohydrates, and healthy fats. Examples include a turkey and cheese sandwich on whole-grain bread, Greek yogurt with berries and nuts, or a protein shake with banana and peanut butter.

- During your workout, stay hydrated by drinking water or a sports drink. You may also want to eat a small snack, such as fruit or a granola bar if you feel hungry or fatigued.

- After your workout, eat a post-workout meal or snack within 30 minutes to an hour. This should be high in protein to help repair and rebuild muscle tissue, and it should also include carbohydrates to replenish glycogen stores. Examples include grilled chicken with sweet potatoes and veggies, a smoothie with protein powder and fruit, or a protein bar with whole-grain crackers.

- Throughout the day, aim to eat small, frequent meals and snacks to keep your energy levels stable and support muscle recovery. Be sure to incorporate plenty of nutrient-dense foods such as lean protein, whole grains, fruits and vegetables, and healthy fats.

It's important to note that individual needs may vary. These are general guidelines that work for most people, but you'll get the best results if you work with a nutrition coach or a registered dietician to develop a personalized nutrition plan tailored to your individual needs and goals.

Hydration

Staying hydrated during the day is just as important as good nutrition. Water is the best hydrator. High-sugar energy drinks will cause your blood sugar levels to spike, after which the levels will crash, leaving you feeling exhausted. Taking good care of your body means cutting down on alcohol, soda, and sugary drinks.

Part of the aging process is the dulling of our sense of thirst. An older person can become dehydrated without feeling very thirsty. Some medications can also increase the risk of dehydration. Inadequate hydration can cause serious health problems, such as urinary tract infections (UTIs), kidney issues, and slower healing from injuries. Make sure you keep hydrated when doing your exercise program.

Hydration is important for strength training for several reasons:

- Optimal muscle function: Our muscles are made up of about 75% water, and dehydration can lead to decreased muscle strength and endurance. This can impair your ability to perform exercises with proper form and limit the amount of weight you can lift.

- Improved performance: When you're dehydrated, your body has to work harder to maintain a safe internal temperature during exercise. This can lead to fatigue and decreased performance, making it harder to complete your strength training routine.

- Faster recovery: Adequate hydration helps your body recover more quickly from intense workouts by replenishing fluids lost during exercise, which helps to reduce muscle soreness and stiffness.

- Injury prevention: Dehydration can increase the risk of injury, such as muscle strains or cramps. Proper hydration helps to maintain the elasticity of muscles and prevent the onset of muscle fatigue.

To ensure that you are properly hydrated for strength training, it is recommended to drink water regularly throughout the day, especially before and after your workout. The amount of water needed will vary depending on the individual, but a good rule of thumb is to aim for at least 8 cups (64 ounces) of water per day. It is also important to note that factors such as exercise intensity, duration, and temperature can increase the amount of water needed to stay properly hydrated.

Sleep

While you are sleeping, your body is recovering from the day's activities. A proper night's rest is essential to give you enough energy for the next day. Sleep problems are an issue for many people. A good workout often leads to better sleep. If you have trouble sleeping, getting regular exercise can help you sleep better, and in turn, better sleep will help you recover from your exercise routine and give you more energy to exercise the next day, creating a beneficial cycle. If you find it difficult to fall asleep, do some night stretches to promote relaxation and wind down from the day.

Sleep is crucial for strength training because the body repairs and rebuilds the muscle tissue that is broken down during exercise as you sleep. When you engage in strength training, your muscles undergo small tears and damage. During the rest and recovery phase, the body repairs the damaged tissue and builds it back stronger and bigger.

A good night's sleep is vital for the body to release growth hormones that help with muscle growth and repair. Lack of sleep can lead to a decrease in growth-hormone production, which can affect muscle growth and recovery.

Furthermore, sleep is critical for energy and focus, which are necessary for an effective workout. Without proper sleep, you may not have the energy or mental clarity to perform your best during strength training sessions, which can compromise your progress.

Overall, getting enough high-quality sleep is essential for optimizing the benefits of strength training, including muscle growth, recovery, and performance. It's recommended to aim for 7–9 hours of sleep per night for most adults to support these goals (Johns Hopkins Medicine, 2019).

Amy's Advice

I am a certified nutrition coach as well as a certified personal trainer. Part of my job is helping clients learn what and how much to eat to keep their bodies healthy. I help them put together a healthy diet that includes each of the macronutrients, carbs, fats, and protein. Most importantly, I teach them an essential lifestyle skill: sticking to healthy habits. Because you can know what to eat, but if you aren't following through with it, then it won't do any good!

What I've found is that people often have an all-or-nothing approach to being healthy. If they can't get their workout in, then they don't have as much of a desire to eat well that day and therefore they don't stay adequately hydrated. On the days they do work out, they find that they eat the rainbow, have plenty of protein, hydrate well with water, and then do their nightly stretches and have a great sleep! The problem is not everyone can tick all the boxes and have the perfect day every day. We want to find a good balance between these habits so that we stick with them! I want to reinforce that you can do some of the healthy habits each day, like get your workout in, drink the water, and stretch—but maybe your meals were off that day and you didn't sleep well. That is okay; keep your goals in mind and try again tomorrow! Because it's not all or nothing. Even taking care of your body by doing three of these healthy things a day is better than doing none.

Chapter 9:
Maintaining Strength and Avoiding Injury

The Importance of Consistency in Strength Training

Consistency is the key to obtaining the full benefits of strength training. If you stick to a regular strength training schedule, you can expect these results:

- Consistent strength training is necessary to build muscle mass. When you strength train, you cause tiny tears in your muscle fibers. Over time, these tears heal and result in increased muscle mass and strength. However, your muscle mass will decrease if you don't strength train regularly.

- Strength training not only builds muscle mass, but also increases strength. Consistent training allows your muscles to adapt and become stronger over time.

- Strength training is also essential for maintaining and improving bone density. As we age, bone density naturally decreases, but strength training can slow down this process.

- Consistent strength training can also boost metabolism, which can help with weight loss or maintenance. Metabolism speeds up because muscle tissue burns more calories at rest than fat tissue.

- Strength training can also help prevent injury by strengthening muscles, tendons, and ligaments. This can improve your balance and stability, reducing the risk of falls and other injuries.

The Importance of Consistency to Maintain Your Exercise Routine

Consistency is crucial when it comes to maintaining an exercise routine. Your whole lifestyle will benefit because consistency results in these rewards:

- When you make exercise a consistent part of your routine, it becomes a habit. This means that it becomes a natural part of your day, and you are more likely to stick with it over the long term.

- Consistent exercise can help you achieve your fitness goals. Whether your goals are losing weight, building muscle, or improving your overall health, regular exercise is essential for making progress.

- Exercise has numerous physical and mental health benefits. It can help lower the risk of chronic diseases, improve cardiovascular health, boost immune function, reduce stress and anxiety, and improve mood and cognitive function. However, these benefits are only achieved through consistent exercise.

- If you halt your exercise routine for an extended period, you may lose the progress you've made. Consistent exercise is essential for maintaining and building on your progress over time.

- Consistency also increases accountability. When you have a consistent exercise routine, you are more likely to hold yourself accountable and make exercise a priority in your life.

Get the Most Out of Your Workout

- Avoid these common exercise pitfalls to get the most out of your workout while reducing the risk of injury or burnout:

- Skipping the warm-up and cool-down can increase the risk of injury and muscle soreness. Take the time to warm up before your workout and cool down afterward to stretch and help your body recover.

- Using improper form during exercises can lead to injury and decrease the effectiveness of the exercise. Make sure to use proper form and technique and ask for guidance from a trainer or coach if needed.

- Overtraining can lead to burnout, injury, and decreased performance. Make sure to incorporate rest days into your workout routine and avoid exercising the same muscle groups on consecutive days.

- It is a smarter strategy to do fewer reps with proper form than more reps with poor form. Focus on quality over quantity to avoid injury and get the best results out of your workout.

- Doing the same workout routine over and over can lead to a plateau in progress and can also become boring. Incorporate variety into your workouts by trying new exercises or changing the intensity, number of reps, or weight.

- Neglecting flexibility and mobility exercises can lead to decreased range of motion and increased risk of injury. Incorporate stretching and mobility exercises into your workout routine to maintain flexibility and mobility.

- Proper nutrition and hydration are essential for optimal performance and recovery. Make sure to fuel your body with the nutrients it needs before and after workouts and stay hydrated throughout the day.

Common Exercise Mistakes That Can Lead to Injury

By avoiding these common exercise mistakes and being mindful of proper technique and safety, you can reduce the risk of injury and make the most out of your workouts. Remember to listen to your body, take rest days when needed, and seek guidance from a professional if you are unsure about proper technique.

- Not warming up: Skipping a proper warm-up before exercise can increase the risk of muscle strain and other injuries.

- Overexertion: Pushing yourself too hard or trying to lift weights that are too heavy can lead to injury.

- Incorrect form: Using incorrect form during exercises can lead to muscle strain, joint pain, and other injuries.

- Not using proper equipment: Using old or worn-out equipment or not using equipment properly can increase the risk of injury.

- Ignoring pain: Ignoring pain during exercise can lead to further injury. If you feel pain during exercise, stop and assess the situation before continuing.

- Doing too much too soon: Trying to do too much too soon can lead to injury, especially if your body is not yet accustomed to the level of activity.

- Neglecting rest and recovery: Overtraining and not allowing enough time for rest and recovery can increase the risk of injury.

Recovery and Rest

Recovery and rest are just as important as the actual workout when it comes to strength training. Proper rest periods are essential to help your body recover from the stresses of exercise and to facilitate the changes in your body you want to see.

Rest for Muscle Repair and Growth

Strength training causes tiny tears in muscle fibers, and recovery time is needed for these muscles to repair and grow stronger. Muscle repair and growth work differently in senior strength training compared to younger adults due to age-related changes in the body. However, anyone of any age can still experience significant improvements in muscle strength and mass with regular strength training. Here's how muscle repair and growth work in senior strength training:

- Muscle damage: When seniors lift weights or perform other resistance exercises, it causes microscopic tears in their muscle fibers. This is normal and necessary for muscle growth and repair.

- Inflammation: After the workout, the body responds to this muscle damage by sending white blood cells to the impacted areas. This causes inflammation, which can lead to soreness and stiffness.

- Repair: Over the next few days, the body repairs the damaged muscle fibers, using protein to create new muscle tissue. This repair process is known as muscle hypertrophy.

- Rest and recovery: The body needs time to recover and build new muscle tissue after strength training. Seniors should allow at least 48 hours of rest between strength training sessions to ensure that their muscles have time to repair and recover.

- Nutrition: Adequate protein intake is essential for muscle repair and growth. Seniors should aim to consume about 1.2–1.5 grams of protein per kilogram of body weight per day to support muscle growth.

Rest for Reduced Risk of Injury

Rest days allow your muscles to recover and reduce the risk of injury from overtraining or fatigue. If you are following a strength training program, rest will protect your body from injury in several ways.

- Recovery time: When you lift weights or perform other resistance exercises, you are placing stress on your muscles, joints, and bones. Rest allows the body time to recover from this stress and repair any damage that may have occurred during the workout. This can help prevent overuse injuries and reduce the risk of acute injuries.

- Joint health: Rest is particularly important for seniors because our joints become more susceptible to wear and tear as we age. By allowing adequate rest between strength training sessions, seniors can give their joints time to recover and reduce the risk of joint injuries.

- Muscle fatigue: Overtraining can cause muscle fatigue, which can increase the risk of injury. If you push yourself too hard and don't allow enough rest between workouts, you may be more likely to experience muscle strains, sprains, or tears.

- Proper form: Rest can also help you maintain proper form during your workouts. As fatigue sets in, it can be more difficult to maintain good technique, which can increase the risk of injury. By taking adequate rest breaks, you can ensure that they are performing each exercise correctly and safely.

In summary, rest is an essential part of any strength training program, particularly for seniors. By allowing adequate time for recovery, we can reduce the risk of injury and maintain good joint and muscle health. You should aim to take at least one day off between strength training sessions and listen to your body if you feel fatigued or in pain.

Rest for Improved Performance

Giving your body time to recover can actually improve your performance in the long run as it allows your muscles to rebuild and become stronger. Your overall performance during your strength training workouts will benefit from adequate rest in the following ways:

- Muscle recovery: When you engage in strength training, your muscles experience micro-tears. Rest allows these tears to repair and the muscles to rebuild, ultimately leading to increased strength and improved performance.

- Energy restoration: Adequate rest between strength training sessions is necessary for restoring energy levels. This can help you maintain your energy levels, which is crucial for optimal performance and motivation.

- Injury prevention: Rest is important for reducing the risk of injury during strength training. Overuse injuries can occur when you engage in strength training without giving your muscles enough time to rest and recover. Injuries will cause you to have to skip workouts, resulting in a loss of progress.

- Mental rejuvenation: Rest is not just beneficial for the body, but also for the mind. Senior strength training can be physically and mentally demanding, so taking time to rest and recover can help seniors feel rejuvenated and motivated to continue their strength training program. If you aren't motivated to continue your program consistently, you are at risk of losing all the exercise benefits you worked hard for.

- Progression: Rest allows the body to adapt to the stresses of strength training and progress to heavier weights or more challenging exercises. Without adequate rest, you may struggle to progress and see improvements in your strength training performance. This can have a negative effect on your goals and motivation.

Rest for Mental Health

Taking rest days can also help with mental health by reducing stress and anxiety associated with overexertion and constantly pushing your body. Your mental health will benefit from proper rest between workouts in the following ways:

- Reducing stress: Senior strength training can be physically and mentally demanding. Adequate rest between strength training sessions can help you reduce stress levels, which can improve mental health and well-being.

- Boosting mood: Rest is important for allowing the body to recover and recharge. This can help you feel more energized and positive, which can boost your mood and overall mental health.

- Preventing burnout: Overtraining can lead to physical and mental burnout, which can have negative effects on mental health. Rest is crucial for preventing burnout and allowing you to continue to be consistent with your strength training program.

- Improving sleep: Rest is essential for allowing the body to recover and rejuvenate, which can improve sleep quality. Improved sleep can have a positive impact on mental health, including reducing symptoms of depression and anxiety.

Rest for Hormonal Balance

Overtraining and lack of rest can disrupt hormonal balance, leading to increased cortisol levels and decreased testosterone levels, which can hinder progress in strength training. Rest is an important aspect of senior strength training that can affect the hormonal balance in the body. Rest can benefit your hormones in the following ways:

- Testosterone: Testosterone is an important hormone for muscle growth and repair. When you engage in strength training, your body releases testosterone to support the growth and repair of muscle tissue. Adequate rest is necessary to allow the body to produce and utilize testosterone effectively. Research has shown that insufficient rest can lead to a drop in testosterone levels, which can impair muscle growth and recovery. (Although testosterone occurs in much higher levels in men and is thus considered a male hormone, women also have testosterone that plays a part in muscle development and repair.) Testosterone levels fall drastically as we age, and our bodies need more time to develop and repair our muscles.

- Cortisol: When we are under stress, our bodies release the stress hormone cortisol. While cortisol is important for maintaining normal bodily functions, excessive cortisol release can have negative effects on muscle growth and recovery. Long periods of exercise without adequate rest can lead to an increase in cortisol levels by increasing the stress on your body. This can result in muscle breakdown, increased risk of injury, and decreased muscle strength.

- Growth hormone: Growth hormone is another hormone that is essential for muscle growth and repair. During rest, the body releases growth hormones to support tissue repair and regeneration. Adequate rest between strength training sessions can help the body produce and utilize growth hormones effectively.

Take care of your body's self-healing needs by giving it the rest and time for recovery it needs. This can mean taking rest days, getting enough sleep, and fueling your body with the right nutrients. Incorporating recovery activities like stretching, foam rolling, and massage can also help with muscle soreness and aid in recovery. Aim for at least one to two rest days per week, and don't be afraid to take more if your body needs it. Be patient. You will see improvements without injury if you take the slow and steady path.

Maintain Your Motivation

To maintain your motivation and keep progressing with your exercise goals, you have to make your workouts a part of your lifestyle. It might be difficult to stay motivated, but there are ways to help you make your strength training a habit.

- Set achievable goals: Set specific and achievable goals for yourself, whether it's increasing the weight you lift or walking a certain distance. It's easier to maintain motivation and focus when you have set clear goals.

- Find an accountability partner: Partnering up with someone who also wants to exercise regularly can help keep you accountable and motivated.

- Schedule your workouts: Treat your workouts like appointments and schedule them into your day. This can help make exercise a priority and ensure that you stick to your routine.

- Mix it up: Doing the same exercise routine over and over can become boring and lead to burnout. Mix up your routines by trying new exercises or activities to keep things fresh and exciting.

- Reward yourself: Celebrate your accomplishments and milestones with rewards that motivate you. This can be something small, like treating yourself to a favorite snack, or something larger, like buying new workout gear.

- Focus on the benefits: Remind yourself of what you stand to gain when you incorporate exercise into your routine, such as improved health, increased energy, and reduced stress. Focusing on these benefits can help keep you motivated to stick to your routine.

- Be flexible: It's okay to miss a workout or have to reschedule. Being flexible and adjusting your routine as needed can help prevent burnout and ensure that you continue to enjoy exercise.

By using these strategies in your routine, you can make exercise a habit and stay motivated to continue with your strength training journey. Remember to start small, be consistent, and celebrate your progress along the way.

Overcoming Time and Energy Challenges

Sometimes, we have too many things going on in our lives for us to stick to our regular routine. We might also look for alternative exercises when our energy levels are low. Being pressed for time or feeling a bit run-down doesn't mean you have to abandon your exercise goals. Here are some ways to help you overcome these challenges:

- Treat exercise as an important part of your daily routine and prioritize it just like you would with work or other responsibilities.

- Plan ahead and schedule your workouts for times when you have the most energy and are least likely to be interrupted.

- Start small and make exercise a daily habit, even if it's just a 10-minute walk or a few simple exercises. As you build consistency, gradually increase the time and intensity of your workouts.

- Look for workouts that are efficient and don't require a lot of time. High-intensity interval training (HIIT) and bodyweight exercises can be great options that can be done in a short amount of time.

- If you are pressed for time, break up your workouts into smaller sessions throughout the day. For example, do 10 minutes of exercise in the morning, afternoon, and evening.

- There are many apps and fitness trackers available that can help you track your workouts and keep you motivated. Use them to set goals, track your progress, and stay on track with your exercise routine.

- Find a workout partner or join a fitness class to help keep you accountable and motivated. Having someone to exercise with can make it more enjoyable and help you stick to your routine.

Remember, even small amounts of exercise can have big benefits for your health and well-being. By overcoming time and energy barriers and making exercise a priority, you can improve your fitness and overall quality of life.

Social Support for Strength Training

There are numerous benefits to working out with a partner or a group. If you struggle with self-discipline, having the support of others can motivate you to stick to your routine. Sometimes it's just more fun to exercise with friends. Laughter and camaraderie make workout days something to look forward to. Here are some of the other benefits of a social support system:

- Motivation: Having a support system can help you stay on track to exercise regularly. Friends or family members who also exercise can provide encouragement and accountability, making it more likely that seniors will stick to their exercise routine.

- Safety: Working out with a partner or in a group can provide an extra layer of safety. If someone experiences dizziness, shortness of breath, or other symptoms during exercise, a workout partner can provide assistance or call for help.

- Enjoyment: Exercising with others can be more enjoyable than working out alone. Socializing during a workout can make it feel less like a boring chore and more like a fun activity.

- Confidence: Seniors who exercise with others may feel more confident in their abilities and less self-conscious about their age or physical limitations. Working out in a supportive environment can help seniors feel more comfortable and confident as they continue to build strength and improve their overall health.

Accountability

It is easier to let our workouts slide if we aren't accountable to a trainer or partner. Without accountability, we might lack the discipline to be consistent with our training. An accountability partner can force us to think about making excuses for skipping a workout. Knowing that someone is expecting you to show up and put in the effort can help you stay committed to your exercise program. If you don't have a partner or a trainer and struggle with self-discipline, you can consider joining an exercise class or an online exercise support group. Exercise classes are run by professionals who have the training to help you with the physical and mental aspects of your workout routine. Your classmates can be a source of support and encouragement as well as accountability partners.

An accountability buddy can help you track your progress over time. A trainer or workout partner can provide feedback on form, technique, and intensity, helping you to gradually increase the difficulty of your workouts and achieve better results. Your exercise partner, trainer, or coach can help you exercise safely and avoid injury. They can monitor your form, provide modifications or alternatives for exercises, and ensure that you are not overexerting yourself. Someone who knows your exercise goals can provide encouragement and support, particularly during challenging workouts or when you are feeling discouraged. This can help you maintain a positive attitude and continue making progress toward your fitness goals.

Consider using a fitness app with community features that allow you to connect with other users, share your progress, and receive support and motivation. Virtual challenges where you pay a small amount to participate will hold you accountable to your wallet. No one likes to waste money.

Chapter 10:
Building Strength and Endurance

Progressive Overload and How to Increase Intensity Gradually

Progressive overload is a basic principle of strength training that involves gradually increasing the stress placed on the muscles over time. The goal of progressive overload is to continually challenge the muscles and force them to adapt and grow stronger.

Here are some ways to apply progressive overload in strength training:

- Increase weight. Gradually increase the amount of weight you lift during your exercises. This can be done by adding more weight to the bar or using heavier dumbbells.

- Increase reps. Do more repetitions of your exercises. This can help improve endurance and muscular strength.

- Increase sets. When you can comfortably do one set, add another set. When you start the new set, do only as many repetitions as you can and gradually add more until you have a full set. This can help increase volume and stimulate muscle growth.

- Decrease rest time. Take less time between sets or exercises. This can help increase the intensity of your workouts and challenge your muscles more.

- Add variety to your routine. Change the exercises you perform to target different muscle groups or to challenge your muscles in new ways.

It's important to remember that progressive overload should be applied gradually and safely to avoid injury. Aim to increase your workload by no more than 10% per week, and listen to your body to avoid overtraining.

Importance of Proper Form

Proper form is important for everyone who engages in strength training, but it is particularly important for seniors. The aging process causes our bodies to become less flexible and more susceptible to injury, so it is essential to use proper form during strength training exercises to minimize the risk of injury.

Here are some reasons why proper form is important for seniors during strength training:

- Correct movement reduces the risk of injury. Using proper form helps minimize the risk of injury, particularly to the joints and muscles. This is especially important for seniors, who are more prone to injury due to age-related changes in the body.

- Doing the movements correctly improves exercise effectiveness. Proper form ensures that the muscles being targeted are being worked effectively, maximizing the benefits of the exercise.

- Proper form helps maintain good posture. Good posture is important for balance and stability, particularly as we age. Proper form during strength training exercises can help seniors maintain good posture and reduce the risk of falls.

- Using proper form helps to improve your range of motion and flexibility, which is important for maintaining mobility and independence as we age.

Incorporating Cardiovascular Exercise to Improve Endurance

The higher your cardiovascular fitness level, the more endurance you will have while exercising. Here are some ways to incorporate cardiovascular exercise into a strength training routine:

- Start with low-impact exercises. When you begin a cardiovascular fitness training program, start with low-impact exercises such as walking, cycling, or swimming, and gradually increase the intensity and duration over time.

- Incorporate interval training into your routine. Interval training is the alternating of periods of high-intensity exercise with periods of rest or low-intensity exercise. This can be incorporated into cardio workouts to increase the intensity and challenge the cardiovascular system.

- Combine strength and cardio exercises. Many strength training exercises can be combined with cardio exercises to create a circuit-style workout that provides both strength and cardiovascular benefits.

- Choose activities that are enjoyable. You are more likely to stick with an exercise routine if you enjoy the activities. Choosing activities that are fun, such as dancing or group fitness classes, can help you stay motivated to reach your goals.

- Try setting a goal to get at least 150 minutes of moderate-intensity cardio exercise each week. The American Heart Association recommends that seniors try to complete at least 150 minutes of moderate-intensity cardio exercise per week, spread out over several days (2021).

Advanced Techniques for Strength Training

Several advanced techniques can be used to help you continue to challenge and improve your strength and fitness over time. Here are some advanced techniques for you to try:

- Plyometrics involves explosive movements that can help improve power and speed. This technique can be incorporated into lower body exercises such as squats or lunges to increase the intensity of the exercise.

- Supersets involve performing two exercises back-to-back without rest. This technique can be used to increase the volume and intensity of a workout while reducing the amount of time required for the workout.

- Isometric exercises involve holding a muscle contraction without movement. This technique can be used to improve strength and stability, particularly in the core and lower body.

- Eccentric training involves focusing on the lowering phase of an exercise, which can help improve strength and muscle size. This technique can be used to target specific muscle groups or to increase the intensity of an exercise.

- Resistance bands can be used to provide additional resistance during strength training exercises, helping to increase the intensity and challenge the muscles. They can also be used to assist with exercises, such as pull-ups, for those who may need additional support.

Plyometric Exercises

Plyometric exercises involve explosive movements that help improve power, speed, and agility. While they may not be appropriate for all seniors, plyometric exercises can be safely incorporated into a strength training program with proper supervision by a certified trainer and modifications. Here are some plyometric exercises that may be suitable to add to your advanced workout:

- Squat jumps: Stand with your feet shoulder-width apart, squat down, then jump up explosively. Land softly and repeat.

- Skater jumps: Start with your feet shoulder-width apart and jump sideways, landing on one foot with the other foot behind you. Jump back to the other side and repeat.

- Box jumps: Stand in front of a sturdy box or step, jump up onto it, then jump back down and repeat.

- Lateral bounds: Stand with your feet shoulder-width apart, then jump sideways as far as you can, landing on one foot with the other foot behind you. Jump back to the starting position and repeat.

- Medicine ball throws: Stand with your feet shoulder-width apart, hold a medicine ball at chest height, and throw it as far as you can to a partner or against a wall. Catch the ball when your partner throws it back or when it bounces back from the wall and repeat.

Plyometric Exercises for the Mobility-Impaired

If you have limited mobility, it's important to discuss your exercise program with your doctor or physical therapist before attempting any plyometric exercises. That being said, here are a few modified plyometric exercises that may be suitable for some individuals with mobility impairments:

- Seated leg extensions: Sit on a chair or wheelchair and place a resistance band around your ankles. Extend one leg out in front of you, pushing against the resistance of the band, then quickly bring it back in. Repeat for 8–10 reps, then switch legs.

- Seated medicine ball slam: Sit on a chair or wheelchair and hold a medicine ball or weighted ball above your head. Quickly slam the ball down onto the ground in front of you, catching it on the rebound. Repeat for 8–10 reps.

- Seated jumping jacks: Sit on a chair or wheelchair and hold a resistance band or hand weights in your hands. Quickly raise your arms up overhead and out to the sides, then bring them back down to your sides. Repeat for 8–10 reps.

- Seated lateral hops: Sit on a chair or wheelchair and place a resistance band around your ankles. Hop your legs out to the side, pushing against the resistance of the band, then quickly bring them back together. Repeat for 8–10 reps.

Remember to start with low repetitions and gradually increase the intensity of your plyometric exercises. It's important to be aware of the limitations of your body and to stop if you experience any pain or discomfort.

Supersets

Supersets can be a useful tool for strength training for seniors as they allow for efficient use of time and can help increase workout intensity. A superset involves performing two exercises in succession with little to no rest in between. Here are some examples of supersets for an advanced training program:

- Upper body superset: Perform 10 repetitions of a seated row exercise immediately followed by 10 reps of a chest press exercise. Rest for 30–60 seconds, then repeat for 2–3 sets.

- Lower body superset: Perform 10 reps of a leg press exercise immediately followed by 10 reps of a calf raise exercise. Rest for 30–60 seconds, then repeat for 2–3 sets.

- Core superset: Perform 10 reps of a plank exercise immediately followed by 8–12 reps of an upper body twist exercise. Rest for 30–60 seconds, then repeat for 2–3 sets.

Supersets for the Mobility-Impaired

If you have mobility difficulties, you don't have to lose out on the benefits of supersets. You can safely do these supersets when sitting on a chair or wheelchair:

- Seated dumbbell curls and tricep extensions: Sit with your spine as straight as you can and hold a dumbbell in each hand. Perform bicep curls with one arm, then immediately perform a tricep extension with the same arm. Do 10 repetitions of each exercise, then switch arms.

- Seated chest press and seated rows: Sit upright and hold a resistance band or hand weights in your hands. Perform a chest press by pushing the weights or band out in front of you, then immediately perform a seated row by pulling the weights or band back toward you. Repeat each exercise 10 times.

- Seated leg extensions and seated leg curls: Place a resistance band around your ankles and sit up straight. Perform leg extensions by extending one leg out in front of you, then immediately perform a leg curl by bending the same leg and bringing your heel toward your glutes. Do 10 extensions and 10 curls, then switch legs.

Remember to start with a weight or resistance level that is appropriate for your strength and gradually increase the intensity as you get stronger. It's important to be aware of your body's limitations and to stop if you experience any pain or discomfort.

Isometric Exercises

Isometric exercises involve holding a muscle in a static contraction without moving the joint. These exercises help improve muscular strength and endurance without putting excessive stress on the joints. Here are some examples of isometric exercises that you might like to try:

- Wall sit: Stand with your back pressed against a wall and slowly lower your body until your knees are bent at a 90-degree angle. Hold this position for 30–60 seconds.

- Plank: Start in a push-up position, then move your forearms to be flat on the ground. Your entire body should be in a straight line from head to heels, engaging your core muscles. Hold for 30–60 seconds.

- Chair pose: Stand with your feet together and slowly lower your glutes into a squat position. Hold your arms straight out in front of you, parallel to the ground. Hold for 30–60 seconds.

- Bridge: Lie down flat and bend your knees so your feet are flat on the ground. Lift your hips up to form a straight line between your shoulders and knees, engaging your glutes and core muscles. Hold for 30–60 seconds.

Isometric Exercises for the Mobility-Impaired

These are some of the isometric exercises that are suitable for an advanced workout if you have limited mobility:

- Wall push-up: Stand facing a wall with your feet shoulder-width apart. Place your palms flat against the wall at chest height and shoulder-width apart. Push against the wall as hard as you can, holding for 10–15 seconds. Rest for 10 seconds, then do 10 more repetitions.

- Seated leg press: Sit on a chair or wheelchair and place your feet flat against a wall or heavy object. Push against the wall or object as hard as you can, holding for 10–15 seconds. Rest for 10 seconds, then repeat the press and hold 10 times.

- Seated abdominal crunch: Sit on a chair or wheelchair and place your hands behind your head. Tighten your abdominal muscles and push your head back against your hands, holding for 10–15 seconds. Rest for 10 seconds, then repeat for 10 reps.

- Seated shoulder press: Sit on a chair or wheelchair and hold weights or resistance bands in your hands. Press the weights or bands up overhead and hold for 10–15 seconds. Rest for 10 seconds, then do 10 more reps.

- Seated calf raise: Sit on a chair or wheelchair with your feet flat on the ground. Push your toes down into the ground as hard as you can and lift your heels, holding for 10–15 seconds. Rest for 10 seconds, and do 10 more repetitions.

When doing isometric contractions, it might be tempting to hold your breath. Do the exercise correctly by remembering to breathe throughout the movements and holds. Holding your breath will raise your blood pressure and can be a serious health risk.

Eccentric Training for Seniors

Eccentric training involves focusing on the lowering or lengthening phase of an exercise, which is when the muscle is lengthening under tension. This type of training can be beneficial for seniors because it helps improve muscle strength and control as well as joint stability. Here are some examples of eccentric exercises that may be suitable for seniors:

- Eccentric squats: Stand with your feet hip-width apart and slowly lower your body down into a squat position. Take 3–5 seconds to lower your body, then stand up quickly. Do 10 of these exercises.

- Eccentric push-ups: Start in a push-up position, then slowly lower yourself down to the ground. Take 3–5 seconds to lower your body, then push yourself back up quickly. Repeat this 10 times.

- Eccentric bicep curls: Hold a dumbbell in each hand with your palms facing up. Curl the weight up toward your shoulders, then slowly lower the weight back down. Take 3–5 seconds to lower the weight, then curl it up quickly. Do 10 repetitions.

Eccentric Exercises for the Mobility-Impaired

Eccentric training is a type of strength training that focuses on the lengthening, or eccentric, phase of muscle contractions. It can be beneficial for improving muscle strength, balance, and mobility in people with mobility impairments. Here are some examples of eccentric training exercises that can be modified for people with limited mobility:

- Seated leg extensions: Sit on a chair or wheelchair and lift one leg up off the ground. Slowly lower it back down to the ground, focusing on the eccentric (lowering) phase of the movement. Do 10 extensions, then switch legs.

- Seated bicep curls: Sit on a chair or wheelchair and hold weights or resistance bands in your hands. Curl your hands up toward your shoulders, then slowly lower them back down, focusing on the eccentric phase of the movement. Perform 10 curls with each arm.

- Seated calf raises: Sit on a chair or wheelchair with your feet flat on the ground. Raise your heels up as high as you can, keeping your toes down, then slowly lower them back down, focusing on the eccentric phase of the movement. Do 10 raises.

- Seated row: Sit on a chair or wheelchair and hold weights or resistance bands in your hands. Pull your elbows back toward your torso, squeezing your shoulder blades together, then slowly release, focusing on the eccentric phase of the movement. Repeat the exercise 10 times.

- Seated shoulder press: Sit on a chair or wheelchair and hold weights or resistance bands in your hands. Press the weights up overhead, then slowly lower them back down, focusing on the eccentric phase of the movement. Do 10 reps.

Remember to move slowly and focus on the eccentric phase of each movement. Don't hold your breath during the movements.

Resistance Band Exercises

Resistance bands are a great tool for senior strength training because they provide a low-impact, joint-friendly way to add resistance to exercises. Here are some resistance band exercises that can help you improve your muscular strength and endurance without aggravating joint pain:

- Seated rows: Sit on a chair with your feet on the ground and loop the resistance band around your feet. Hold the ends of the band with your hands, then pull the band toward your body, squeezing your shoulder blades together. Slowly release and repeat for a set of 10 reps.

- Chest press: Lie down flat with your knees bent and loop the resistance band around your back. Hold the ends of the band and then press the band away from your body until your arms are straight. Move your arms back slowly. Do 10 chest presses.

- Leg press: Sit on a chair with your feet flat on the ground and loop the resistance band around your feet. Hold the ends of the band, then press your feet out against the resistance of the band. Bring your feet back slowly and do a set of 10 reps.

- Bicep curls: Stand on the resistance band with your feet hip-width apart and hold the ends of the band with your hands. Curl the band up toward your shoulders, then slowly move your arms back to the starting position. Do a set of 10 curls.

High-Intensity Interval Training

High-intensity interval training (HIIT) can be a great option if you want to improve your cardiovascular fitness and overall health. HIIT is a type of exercise where you alternate periods of high-intensity exercise with periods of rest or low-intensity exercise. Here are some of the many benefits HIIT can provide for seniors:

- Increased cardiovascular fitness. HIIT is an effective way to develop cardiovascular fitness in people of all ages, including seniors.

- Time-efficient workouts. HIIT workouts can be completed in a relatively short amount of time, making them a great option if you have limited time or may not be able to tolerate longer periods of exercise.

- Improved insulin sensitivity. HIIT has been shown to counteract insulin insensitivity, which is important for seniors who may be at risk for diabetes or other metabolic conditions.

- Increased muscle strength and endurance. HIIT workouts can be designed to target specific muscle groups, which can help you maintain and improve your muscle strength and endurance.

HIIT Exercises for Seniors

High-intensity interval training is an effective way for seniors to improve their cardiovascular health, balance, and overall fitness. You can begin to include these exercises in your workout routine and add more time as your endurance increases:

- Walking or jogging intervals: Start with a brisk walk for 30 seconds, then increase the pace to a light jog for 30 seconds. Aim to keep this up for 5 minutes.

- Cycling intervals: Start with a slow pace for 30 seconds, then increase the resistance and speed for 30 seconds. Try to do this for at least 5 minutes.

- Chair squats: Sit on a chair with your feet hip-width apart. Stand up and sit back down repeatedly for 30 seconds, then rest for 30 seconds. If you are a beginner, work toward completing a 5-minute session.

- Modified jumping jacks: Start by standing with your feet together and arms at your sides. Jump your feet out to shoulder-width apart while raising your arms above your head, then jump back to the starting position. If jumping is too challenging, step one foot out at a time instead. Repeat the jumps for 30 seconds, then rest for 30 seconds. Repeat this sequence for 5 minutes.

- Step-ups: Stand in front of a step or sturdy bench. Step up with one foot, then step the other foot up next to it. Step back down with one foot, then the other. Repeat for 30 seconds leading with one leg, then switch to the other leg for 30 seconds. Rest for 30 seconds, then repeat for 5 minutes.

HIIT for the Mobility-Impaired

High-intensity interval training exercises may not be suitable for everyone, especially those with mobility impairments. However, there are modified HIIT exercises that can be performed by people with limited mobility. Here are some examples:

- Seated knee lifts: Sit on a chair or wheelchair and lift one knee up toward your chest as high as you can. Lower it back down and repeat with the other leg. Repeat this for 30–60 seconds.

- Seated arm curls: Sit on a chair or wheelchair and hold weights or resistance bands in your hands. Curl your arms up toward your shoulders and slowly lower them back down. Aim for 30–60 seconds.

- Seated marching: Sit on a chair or wheelchair and lift one foot up off the ground, then lower it back down and repeat with the other leg. Alternate legs for 30–60 seconds.

- Seated torso twists: Sit on a chair or wheelchair with your feet flat on the ground. Twist your torso to the right, then twist to the left. Alternate the direction of the twist for 30–60 seconds.

- Seated jumping jacks: Sit on a chair or wheelchair and lift both arms up over your head. At the same time, kick both legs out to the side, then bring them back in and lower your arms. Repeat for 30–60 seconds.

Overcoming Plateaus in Strength Training

You might find that at a certain stage in your training, you stop seeing progress despite being consistent with your program. Plateaus in strength training can be frustrating, but they are a normal part of the training process. Overcoming plateaus requires a strategic approach that involves making changes to your training program to challenge your body in new ways. Here are some tips for overcoming plateaus in strength training:

- Change your exercises. If you've been doing the same exercises for a while, your body may have adapted to the movements, and you may no longer be challenging your muscles enough. Switching up your exercises can help you target different muscle groups and challenge your body in new ways.

- Increase your weight or resistance. Gradually increasing the weight or resistance you use during your exercises can help you continue to challenge your muscles and break through plateaus.

- Vary your sets and reps. Changing the number of sets and reps you perform can help you challenge your muscles in different ways. For example, increasing the number of reps you perform can help improve muscular endurance, while decreasing the number of reps and increasing the weight can help improve muscular strength.

- Incorporate new training techniques. Incorporating techniques such as supersets, HIIT, or eccentric training can challenge your muscles in new ways and help you overcome plateaus.

- Ensure adequate rest and recovery. Overtraining can lead to plateaus and even injury. Make sure you're taking enough time for your body to recover between workouts and consider incorporating rest days or active recovery activities into your routine.

Remember, breaking through plateaus requires patience, consistency, and dedication to your training program. By making strategic changes to your program and focusing on proper form and technique, you can continue to make progress in your strength training journey.

Using Wii for Strength Training

Using a Nintendo Wii for senior strength training can be a fun and effective way to develop your strength, balance, and overall fitness. Wii Fit and Wii Sports are two popular games that can be used for strength training.

Here are some benefits of using Wii for senior strength training:

- The movements used in Wii games are low-impact and easy on the joints, making them ideal if you have mobility issues or are recovering from an injury.

- The Wii Fit game includes a body test feature that assesses the player's balance, body mass index (BMI), and other fitness measures. The game then creates a personalized workout plan based on the results of the body test.

- Wii Fit includes a variety of strength training exercises, such as squats, lunges, and arm curls, as well as balance exercises like yoga and balance games. This variety helps to keep the workouts interesting and engaging.

- The game's scoring system and virtual rewards can be motivating for seniors, encouraging them to work harder and stay engaged with the workout.

- Seniors can do Wii workouts from the comfort of their own homes, making it a convenient and accessible option for those who may not be able to make it to a gym or community center.

If you want to add something new to your workouts with Wii, remember that you should still include warm-ups and cool-downs to prevent injury.

Future Directions in Strength Training for Seniors

Strength training for seniors has come a long way in recent years, and there are several exciting trends and developments that are shaping the future of this field. Here are some potential future directions in strength training for seniors:

- Technology-assisted training. Developing technologies such as virtual reality, augmented reality, and wearable devices are becoming more common in the fitness industry, and there is potential for these tools to be used in strength training for seniors. Virtual reality, for example, can be used to simulate real-world activities and provide an interactive training experience. With virtual reality, you can enjoy being out on the golf course and working on your swing without leaving your living room.

- Personalized training programs. As more data becomes available about individual seniors' health and fitness, there is potential for more personalized training programs to be developed. These programs take into account individual factors such as health status, fitness level, and personal goals. With the current advances in biotechnology, it is possible that training programs will be tailored to your unique needs via DNA analysis.

- Multimodal training programs. Combining different types of exercise, such as strength training, cardiovascular exercise, and balance training, can be an effective way to improve overall fitness and reduce the risk of falling and other injuries. Multimodal training programs that incorporate a variety of exercises could become more common in the future.

- Emphasis on functional training. Functional training focuses on exercises that mimic real-world activities and movements, and there is growing interest in this type of training for seniors. Functional training can help seniors maintain their independence and improve their ability to perform activities of daily living.

- Focus on cognitive health. Exercise has been shown to improve cognitive health, and there is potential for strength training to be used specifically to improve cognitive function in seniors. Future research could explore the potential cognitive benefits of strength training and develop targeted training programs.

- Virtual and online fitness classes: With the rise of at-home workouts due to the COVID-19 pandemic, virtual and online fitness programs have become increasingly popular.

Many gyms and fitness studios now offer virtual classes and personal training sessions, and there are also numerous online fitness programs and apps available.

- Wearable technology: Technology that you can wear on your body such as fitness trackers, smartwatches, and heart rate monitors has become ubiquitous in the fitness industry. These devices provide users with valuable data about their workouts and can help motivate them to stay active. The information about your heart rate, duration of exercise, number of steps taken, and calories burnt can be kept on your computer or on your wearable, making it easy to track your progress.

- Health and wellness coaching: Employing the services of health and wellness coaches has become more prevalent in the fitness industry as people seek guidance and support in achieving their health and fitness goals. Coaches can help individuals with everything from nutrition to mindset and goal setting. Life coaches and motivational speakers can add their expertise to the fitness industry and help develop their clients' self-discipline and consistency.

Overall, the future of strength training for seniors is bright, and there are many exciting opportunities for research, innovation, and new developments in this field.

The Future of Strength Training for the Mobility-Impaired

As life expectancy increases, there is an increasing need for effective and accessible strength training programs for people with mobility impairments. Here are some potential future directions for strength training for this population:

- Personalized training programs. As technology advances, there is potential for the development of personalized strength training programs that take into account an individual's specific mobility impairment, strength level, and other factors. This could help to optimize outcomes and reduce the risk of injury.

- Virtual reality and gaming. Virtual reality and gaming technologies could be used to make strength training more engaging and enjoyable for people with mobility impairments. This could also help to improve adherence to exercise programs.

- Group exercise programs. Group exercise programs have been shown to be effective in improving strength and mobility in older adults. There is potential for the development of group strength training programs that are specifically designed for people with mobility impairments.

- Combining strength training with other interventions. There is potential for combining strength training with other interventions, such as balance training, gait training, and cognitive training, to improve overall mobility and quality of life in people with mobility impairments.

- Focus on community-based programs. Community-based programs can be effective in improving strength and mobility in older adults. There is potential for the development of community-based strength training programs that are specifically designed for people with mobility impairments, which could improve accessibility and engagement.

The future of strength training for people with mobility impairments is promising, and there is potential for continued advancements in the field to improve outcomes and quality of life.

Strength Training Games for Seniors

Strength training games can be a fun and engaging way for seniors to improve their strength and overall fitness. Here are some examples of strength training games for seniors:

- Balloon volleyball: Inflate a balloon and use it to play a volleyball game. This game can help improve upper body strength, coordination, and endurance.

- Chair squats: Place a chair against a wall and have seniors sit down and stand up from the chair repeatedly. This exercise can help improve leg strength.

- Resistance band tug-of-war: Divide seniors into teams and have them play a game of tug-of-war using resistance bands. This game can help improve upper body strength and endurance.

- Ball toss: Have seniors toss a medicine ball or weighted ball back and forth with a partner. This game can help improve upper body strength and coordination.

- Bodyweight bingo: Create a bingo card with different bodyweight exercises, such as planks, squats, lunges, and push-ups. Seniors can play a game of bingo by performing the exercises on the card.

Remember to choose exercises and games that are appropriate for the abilities and fitness level of everyone participating. Always prioritize safety and encourage participants to listen to their bodies and take breaks as needed.

Strength Training Sports for Seniors

Strength training sports can be a great way for seniors to improve their strength, endurance, balance, and overall fitness while having fun and enjoying a social activity. Below are some strength training sports for seniors:

- Pickleball is a low-impact sport that can be played indoors or outdoors. It combines elements of tennis, badminton, and ping-pong and can help improve hand-eye coordination, balance, and cardiovascular fitness.

- Bowling is a great way to improve upper body strength and endurance as well as balance and coordination.

- Golf is a low-impact sport that can help improve strength, flexibility, and balance. Walking the course and carrying your clubs can also provide a cardiovascular workout.

- Tai chi is a specialized form of martial arts that involves slow, controlled movements and can help improve balance, flexibility, and strength.

- Aquatic exercises, such as water aerobics, can be a great way to improve strength and endurance while minimizing stress on your joints.

Aquatic Strength Training

Aquatic strength training can be a fun way to increase your strength, endurance, and overall fitness in a low-impact environment. The risk of injury is lower than with regular exercises, making aquatic exercises a suitable alternative for beginners who are very frail. Exercising in water reduces the load on joints, making it ideal for people with joint pain or who are recovering from injuries. An added bonus is that it is easier to build strength in water because water offers more resistance to movement than air. Here are some examples of aquatic strength training exercises:

- Walking in water provides resistance that can help improve leg strength and endurance. Seniors can walk forward, backward, and sideways in chest-deep water.

- Water aerobics classes offer a full-body workout that can help improve strength, flexibility, and cardiovascular fitness. Exercises can include arm curls, leg lifts, and twists.

- Seniors can use foam dumbbells or resistance bands in the water to perform strength training exercises for the upper body.

- Pool noodles can be used as a resistance tool for exercises such as leg lifts, bicycle kicks, and core twists.

- Running in deep water with a buoyancy belt can provide a low-impact cardiovascular workout that can also help improve leg strength.

Conclusion

If you invest in your body, you are investing in your future quality of life. If you dedicate yourself to a strength training program, you are investing in your physical independence. This book has given you the tools to build a healthy lifestyle that will make your senior years more active and enjoyable.

It is never too late—or too early—to start. Your body is a magnificent machine capable of self-healing and self-improving. You can gain muscle strength, flexibility, and bone density through your lifestyle. Being more capable of doing everyday tasks will boost your confidence and self-esteem.

Being consistent and chasing your goals of a healthy lifestyle will reward you with well-deserved pride in your achievements. Your energy levels will increase and your stamina will improve. Activities that you might have given up will become enjoyable again. Your joints will become looser and your blood pressure lower. You will live without the constant fear of falling and worrying about broken hips and shattered wrists.

You don't have to wish for or imagine what a stronger body and healthier lifestyle can do for you. You can make it a reality and see for yourself. It is a journey where every destination leads to a new goal. Strength training is an adventure, and it is fun.

The best part? A healthy lifestyle is easy to achieve. You don't have to deprive yourself of the occasional treat or force yourself to drink expensive concoctions that promise you health in a glass. You can reach your fitness goals by using only your body, a chair, and something that will offer resistance to movement, such as a kettlebell, a set of dumbbells, or a resistance band. If you have mobility issues, you can do the modified exercises and feel the positive difference in your body and mindset. You CAN do it.

If you want to connect with me, find me at:
amynealcoaching.com

or on Facebook at:
Amy Neal Coaching

Thank you for reading Strength Training for Seniors!

If you enjoyed this book, I'd appreciate it
if you'd leave a review on Amazon!

Reviews help independent writers, like me,
get my book into the hands of more people like you!

I have provided a link that will take you directly to my review page!
You can copy and paste it directly into the search bar on your computer.
Or click the live link from the device you are reading!

Thank you, again for reading my book.
Stay strong and healthy!

https://mybook.to/yzKO

References

Alzheimer's Society. (2019). *Physical exercise and dementia.* Alzheimer's Society. https://www.alzheimers.org.uk/about-dementia/risk-factors-and-prevention/physical-exercise

American Heart Association. (2021). *The American Heart Association's diet and lifestyle recommendations.* Www.heart.org. https://www.heart.org/en/healthy-living/healthy-eating/eat-smart/nutrition-basics/aha-diet-and-lifestyle-recommendations

The anti-aging effects of exercise. (2018, April 15). Michigan Today. https://michigantoday.umich.edu/2018/04/15/the-anti-aging-effects-of-exercise/

Arnarson, A. (2017, February 16). *The fat-soluble vitamins: A, D, E and K.* Healthline. https://www.healthline.com/nutrition/fat-soluble-vitamins

Best chair exercises for seniors: Safe and easy workouts. (2022, October 31). Www.medicalnewstoday.com. https://www.medicalnewstoday.com/articles/chair-exercises-for-seniors

Cat/cow pose. (n.d.). Mayo Clinic. https://www.mayoclinic.org/healthy-lifestyle/stress-management/multimedia/cat-cow-pose/vid-20453581

Centers for Disease Control and Prevention. (2021, November 1). *Benefits of physical activity.* CDC.gov. https://www.cdc.gov/physicalactivity/basics/pa-health/index.htm

Child's pose. (n.d.). Mayo Clinic. https://www.mayoclinic.org/healthy-lifestyle/stress-management/multimedia/childs-pose/vid-20453580

Cronkleton, E. (2019, July 15). *Chest press: How to, benefits, variations, and more.* Healthline. https://www.healthline.com/health/exercise-fitness/chest-press

Davis, N. (2019, November 21). *How to do a Bulgarian split squat—And why you should.* Healthline. https://www.healthline.com/health/fitness-exercise/bulgarian-split-squat

DOMS: *Prevention and treatment of delayed-onset muscle soreness.* (2006, November 30). BodyBuilding.com. https://www.bodybuilding.com/content/doms-prevention-and-treatment-of-delayed-onset-muscle-soreness.html

Everything you've ever wanted to know about muscles. (n.d.). Popular Science. https://www.popsci.com/build-muscle-faq-exercise-experts/

Exercises for people with limited mobility and physical disability. (2022, January 5). Ultrahuman. https://ultrahuman.com/blog/exercises-for-people-limited-mobility-physical-disability/

4 HIIT workouts for seniors that prove it's really possible—Loaids. (n.d.). Elizabeth. https://surebonus.mystrikingly.com/blog/4-hiit-workouts-for-seniors-that-prove-it-s-really-possible-loaids

Freedman, V. A., & Martin, L. G. (1998). Understanding trends in functional limitations among older Americans. *American Journal of public health, 88*(10), 1457–1462. https://doi.org/10.2105/ajph.88.10.1457

Freutel, N. (2020, March 5). *5 joint mobility exercises to improve flexibility and function.* Healthline. https://www.healthline.com/health/fitness-exercise/joint-mobility-exercises

Harvard Health Publishing. (2021, February 15). *Exercise can boost your memory and thinking skills.* Harvard Health. https://www.health.harvard.edu/mind-and-mood/exercise-can-boost-your-memory-and-thinking-skills

Healthy aging begins with muscles. (2017, December 15). Exercise Coach. https://exercisecoach.com/the-anti-aging-effect-of-strength-training/

HIIT for seniors [Read this before trying]. (2019, January 30). Elder Strength. https://elderstrength.com/hiit-for-seniors/

How can strength training build healthier bodies as we age? (n.d.). National Institute on Aging. https://www.nia.nih.gov/news/how-can-strength-training-build-healthier-bodies-we-age

How to be consistent and why it's important to your success. (n.d.). Www.morningcoach.com. https://www.morningcoach.com/blog/how-to-be-consistent-and-why-it-s-important-to-your-success

Hurst, C., Robinson, S. M., Witham, M. D., Dodds, R. M., Granic, A., Buckland, C., De Biase, S., Finnegan, S., Rochester, L., Skelton, D. A., & Sayer, A. A. (2022). Resistance exercise as a treatment for sarcopenia: prescription and delivery. *Age and aging, 51*(2). https://doi.org/10.1093/ageing/afac003

The importance of hydration during exercise. (2020, October 30). Australian Fitness Academy. https://www.fitnesseducation.edu.au/blog/health/the-importance-of-hydration-during-exercise/

Johns Hopkins Medicine. (2019). *Exercising for better sleep.* Johns Hopkins Medicine. https://www.hopkinsmedicine.org/health/wellness-and-prevention/exercising-for-better-sleep

Kamb, S. (2019, September 22). *Bodyweight dip 101 (How to perform the dip exercise) | Nerd Fitness.* https://www.nerdfitness.com/blog/how-to-do-a-perfect-dip-no-tobacco-required/

Kettlebell swings: Benefits and how to do them right. (2022, January 28). Healthline. https://www.healthline.com/health/fitness/benefits-of-kettle-bell-swings

LaMotte, S. (2022, October 17). *Look to exercise to extend life, even for the oldest, study says.* CNN. https://www.cnn.com/2022/10/17/health/strength-training-live-longer-wellness/index.html

Marturana Winderl, A. (2019, March 7). *What functional training is and why it's important.* SELF. https://www.self.com/story/what-functional-training-is-why-its-important

Mayo Clinic Staff. (2021, January 15). *7 Tips to help you stick with your fitness Program.* Mayo Clinic. https://www.mayoclinic.org/healthy-lifestyle/fitness/in-depth/fitness/art-20047624

McKenna, J. (n.d.). *Weight training and cholesterol.* WebMD. https://www.webmd.com/cholesterol-management/weight-training-cholesterol

Mills, M. (2020, January 28). *18 chair exercises for seniors & how to get started.* Vive Health. https://www.vivehealth.com/blogs/resources/chair-exercises-for-seniors

The national council on aging. (2021, August 23). Www.ncoa.org. https://www.ncoa.org/article/how-to-stay-hydrated-for-better-health/

Nitschke, E. (2018, November 29). *Proper form for a one-arm dumbbell row.* National Federation of Professional Trainers. https://www.nfpt.com/blog/proper-form-for-a-one-arm-dumbbell-row

Nordqvist, J. (2021, January 4). *Vitamin C: Why we need it, sources, and how much is too much.* Www.medicalnewstoday.com. https://www.medicalnewstoday.com/articles/219352

Perry, M., CSCS, & CPT. (2020, September 15). *How to do a reverse lunge with proper form & technique.* Www.builtlean.com. https://www.builtlean.com/reverse-lunge-exercise/

Quinn, E. (2007, May 22). *Why athletes need rest and recovery after exercise.* Verywell Fit; Verywellfit. https://www.verywellfit.com/the-benefits-of-rest-and-recovery-after-exercise-3120575

Quinn, E. (2019). *The basic bridge exercise for core stability.* Verywell Fit. https://www.verywellfit.com/how-to-do-the-bridge-exercise-3120738

Reddy, P., & Jialal, I. (2020). *Biochemistry, vitamin, fat soluble.* PubMed; StatPearls Publishing. https://www.ncbi.nlm.nih.gov/books/NBK534869/

Robinson, L., & Segal, J. (2019). *How to exercise with limited mobility.* HelpGuide.org. https://www.helpguide.org/articles/healthy-living/chair-exercises-and-limited-mobility-fitness.htm

Russ, M. (2005, August 12). *Consistency: The most important element of training.* ACTIVE.com. https://www.active.com/fitness/articles/consistency-the-most-important-element-of-training

Sarcopenia (muscle loss): Symptoms & causes. (2022, June 3). Cleveland Clinic. https://my.clevelandclinic.org/health/diseases/23167-sarcopenia

Schultz, R. (2019, May 10). *This single move targets your butt, legs, and core.* Women's Health. https://www.womenshealthmag.com/fitness/a27423100/single-leg-deadlift-exercise/

The side-bend stretch: A gentle exercise. (n.d.). Www.urmc.rochester.edu. https://www.urmc.rochester.edu/encyclopedia/content.aspx?contenttypeid=1&contentid=4469

Six trends in strength training. (2018, May 12). SPLITFIT. https://splitfit.com/personal-training/six-trends-in-strength-training/

Stoneham, A. (2020, February 18). *6 essential functional movements.* Body Glide. https://www.bodyglide.com/blog/6-essential-functional-movements/

Streit, L. (2018, September 27). *Micronutrients: Types, functions, benefits and more.* Healthline. https://www.healthline.com/nutrition/micronutrients

Streit, L. (2021, November 1). *What are macronutrients? All you need to know.* Healthline. https://www.healthline.com/nutrition/what-are-macronutrients

Strength training for seniors: Everything you need to know. (2019, May 13). SilverSneakers. https://www.silversneakers.com/blog/strength-training-for-seniors/

Taylor, S. (2020, October 13). *Warm up for injury prevention and performance.* The Center Foundation. https://www.centerfoundation.org/warm-up-for-injury-prevention/

13 benefits of strength training for people older than 50. (n.d.). Human Kinetics. https://us.humankinetics.com/blogs/articles/13-benefits-of-strength-training-for-people-older-than-50

Thurman, C. D., Joey. (n.d.). *How to stretch hamstrings and prevent injury in 7 easy ways.* Insider. https://www.insider.com/guides/health/fitness/hamstring-stretch

A 20-minute seated strength workout for anyone with limited mobility. (n.d.). LIVESTRONG.COM. https://www.livestrong.com/article/13726091-seated-strength-workout-limited-mobility/

20 plank exercises that will seriously strengthen your abs. (n.d.). Health.com. https://www.health.com/fitness/20-plank-exercises-you-can-do-at-home

V-Sits improve balance and core stability—Here's what you need to know. (n.d.). Byrdie. https://www.byrdie.com/v-sit-5179839

Waehner, P. (n.d.). *How to avoid a plateau with progressive resistance.* Verywell Fit. https://www.verywellfit.com/progressive-resistance-1229835

Why you should start doing planks. (2021, November 18). Cleveland Clinic. https://health.clevelandclinic.org/plank-exercise-benefits/

Williams, L. (2021, December 8). *Develop shoulder strength with the side lateral raise exercise.* Verywell Fit. https://www.verywellfit.com/side-lateral-raise-4588211

Printed in Great Britain
by Amazon